KETO AIR FRYER COOKBOOK

Delicious Low-carb Air Fryer Recipes to Lose Weight Rapidly

(Grill and Roast With Your Air Frye)

Jose Renfro

Published by Sharon Lohan

© **Jose Renfro**

All Rights Reserved

Keto Air Fryer Cookbook: Delicious Low-carb Air Fryer Recipes to Lose Weight Rapidly (Grill and Roast With Your Air Frye)

ISBN 978-1-990334-00-9

All rights reserved. No part of this guide may be reproduced in any form without permission in writing from the publisher except in the case of brief quotations embodied in critical articles or reviews.

Legal & Disclaimer

The information contained in this book is not designed to replace or take the place of any form of medicine or professional medical advice. The information in this book has been provided for educational and entertainment purposes only.

The information contained in this book has been compiled from sources deemed reliable, and it is accurate to the best of the Author's knowledge; however, the Author cannot guarantee its accuracy and validity and cannot be held liable for any errors or omissions. Changes are periodically made to this book. You must consult your doctor or get professional medical advice before using any of the suggested remedies, techniques, or information in this book.

Table of contents

Part 1 1

Introduction 2

Chapter One: Living a Clean Keto Lifestyle 3

Chapter Two: What's Keto Diet 4

How does the Keto work? 4

Ketosis 7

Benefits of Keto Diet 8

How to Lose Weight with the Ketogenic Diet? 10

Foods to Avoid On Keto Diet 13

Keto Pantry Essential 16

Chapter Three: What is an Air Fryer? 18

The Benefits of Air Fryer 19

Step-By-Step Air Frying 21

Uses of an Air Fryer 22

Good Fats That Are Suitable for Air Frying 23

Chapter Four: Keto Dairy Free Air Fryer Recipe 26

August Liver Burger 26

Sesame Salad with Beef Strips 27

Stuffed Beef Heart 30

Whole Chicken with Rosemary 31

Juicy Keto Turkey Rolls 33

Keto Chicken Breast 34

Indian Lamb Meatballs 35

Pork Chops with Keto Gravy 37

Keto Sandwich (Bread-Free) 39

Winter Squash Tots 40

Spiced Cucumber Chips 41

Bacon Omelet 42

Keto Fish Fries 43

Mushroom Omelet 45

Shredded Beef with Herbs 47

Beef Strips with Zucchini Spirals 48

Chapter Five: Keto Air Fryer Weight Loss Recipes 51

Keto Chinese Greens 51

Turnip Mash 52

Air Fryer Creamy Snow Peas 53

Keto Summer Vegetables 54

Liver Pate 56

Flax Meal Porridge 57

Keto-Jerk Chicken Wings 58

Toasted Nuts 60

Keto Nuggets 61

Eggplant Chips	62
Winter Squash Tots	63
Spiced Cucumber Chips	64
Beef Strips with Zucchini Spirals	65
Stuffed Beef Heart	67
Whole Chicken with Rosemary	68
Juicy Keto Turkey Rolls	69
Swedish Meatballs	71
Turmeric Cauliflower Rice	73
Spiced Asparagus	75
Sriracha Broccoli	76
Blackberry Muffins	78
Egg Soufflé	79
Wrapped Bacon Asparagus	80
Buffalo Cauliflower	82
Hemp Seeds Porridge	83
Parsley Coconut Butter Mushrooms	84
Keto Crab Mushrooms	87
Bacon Cabbage	88
Garlic Zucchini Pate	89
Chapter Six: Air Fryer Gluten-Free Recipes	91
Onion Rings	91

Crispy Tofu	92
Mushroom & risotto chorizo balls	93
Orange Sesame Chicken	95
Banana Chips	96
Egg & Potato Breakfast Platter	97
Cheesy Bacon Quiche	98
Karaage Chicken	100
Crisped Calamari	101
Choco-Banana Cake	103
Crispy Garlic	104
Shrimps with Spicy Orange Marmalade	105
Turkey Meatballs	106
Buffalo Meat balls	107
Chicken Nuggets	108
Almond Flavored Chicken Nuggets	108
Crispy Polenta	109
Roasted Pork Ribs	110
Sweet & Sour Pork	112
Baked Crayfish	113
Garlic Butter Clams	114
Tuna Cutlets	115
Cheesy Spicy Paneer Patties	116

Quinoa Broccoli Fritters	117
Lamb Meatballs	118
Fish & Chips	118
Cheese Straws	119
Crisped Broccoli	120
Chicken Wings	121
Potato-Plantain Kebabs	123
Tandoori Chicken	124
Chapter Seven: Air Fryer Vegan Recipes	126
Turmeric Potato Chips	126
Spinach Potato Kebabs	127
Avocado Fries	128
Apple Chips	129
Rice Stuffed Tomatoes	129
Breakfast Burritos	130
Cauliflower Fried Rice	132
Fish Taco Wraps	133
Vegan Balls	134
Sweet Potato Popcorn	135
Stuffed Bell Pepper	136
Spiced Peanuts	137
Khichdi Balls	138

Chickpea Samosa 139

Sago Carrot Cutlets 140

Corn Vadas 141

Lemon Flavored Green Beans 142

Crispy Spanish Potatoes 144

Baked Tofu Fingers 145

Crispy Kale 146

Chapter Eight: Air Fryer Low-Carb Recipes 147

Cheesy Paneer Patties 147

Creamy Crispy Paneer Kebabs 148

Fried Aubergine 149

Stuffed Mushrooms 150

Cauliflower Steak 150

Stuffed Crab 151

Cheesy Scrambled Eggs 153

Chicken in Screw Pine Leaves 154

Tilapia Salad 155

Spicy Chicken Wings 155

Prawns in Creamy Garlic Sauce 156

Roasted Pork belly 157

Crispy Kale 158

Cheesy Broccoli 159

Salmon with Almond Crust 160

Balsamic Broccoli 160

Beef Steak 161

Mini Lamb Rump Roast 162

Lamb Chops 163

Balsamic Brussels Sprouts 164

Cajun Seasoned Salmon 165

Garlic Flavored Mushroom 165

Cauliflower Bites 166

Shrimps Wrapped in Bacon 168

Veggie Mix 168

Conclusion 170

Part 2 171

Baked Avocado Egg 171

Scotch Eggs with Spicy Pepper Sauce 173

Easy Frittata Breakfast 175

White Bean Toasts with Burst Grape Tomatoes and Pancetta 176

Loaded Cauliflower Hashbrowns 179

Deep Dish Prosciutto, Spinach & Mushroom Pizza - Air Fryer Version 182

Monte Cristo Sandwich 185

Keto Creamed Spinach 187

Part 1

Introduction

Most people find it difficult to live a clean keto lifestyle, but that's one of the easiest things to achieve if one is determined and dedicated. Living a clean keto life and mastering it is very easy, convenient and delicious, but you need to know the basics which includes how and why the diets works, the benefits and the best ways to make it a lasting lifestyle.

An air fryer as we all know is a cooking appliance which helps to cook various delicious and tasty dishes at home. Air fryer cooks food by circulating hot air into an air fryer chamber. This is a device where you can fry something like French fries with a little oil and that's one of the benefits of this device called Air Fryer device as it save up to 80 percent of oil while frying or cooking food. People do complain of lack of crispiness in their food, air fryer makes your food crispy you guys don't need to worry about that again.

Clean Keto Air-fryer Cookbook is a book that gives you every detail on how to live and maintain clean keto lifestyle, how to engage yourself with keto diet, All you need to know about your air-fryer device and the last but not the least over 500 Dairy-Free, Gluten-Free, Paleo, Whole, Plant-base, Nut-Free, Sugar-Free, Soy-Free, Grain-Free Recipe For Allergy Based Weight loss And Healing.

Chapter One: Living a Clean Keto Lifestyle

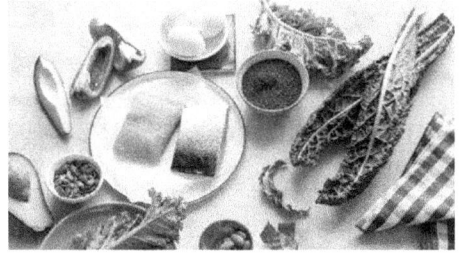

Most people find it difficult to live a clean keto lifestyle, but that's one of the easiest things to achieve if one is determined and dedicated. Living a clean keto life and mastering it is very easy, convenient and delicious, but you need to know the basics which includes how and why the diets works, the benefits and the best ways to make it a lasting lifestyle.

You don't need to panic, as I have got you covered. On this chapter, I will be able to break it down so that you will be able to put it into practice immediately.

Sharing information with people have been path of me for years and am very happy with the testimonies people came back to share with me after going through some of my works on my websites. Every information in this book is detailed; you will be able to digest it well whether you know much about keto or a newbie.

Chapter Two: What's Keto Diet

Am cutting straight to the chase

Keto diet is simply a low-carb diet burns fuel from fat in the body instead of carbohydrates. It allows you to shed weight efficiently, enjoy and endless source of energy and carves the body into the best state of heath both physically and mentally.

Unlike other low carb diets, you don't stuff yourself with processed foods, unhealthy fried foods and all the junk your body craves, which you know are not good for you.

Keto diet is more like eating whole foods, which are very close to their pure state as possible, just like nature intended. It's like going back to the basics and enjoying real food.

Engaging yourself with keto diet will not make you to deprive yourself food whenever you are hungry, it's all about healing your destructive relationship with food i.e eating only healthy fun stuff that boast yourself image and make you fall in love with exciting food all over again just as you are made to be.

How does the Keto work?

Our body has two fuel sources, the glucose which is created by your body from the carbohydrate that you eat in grains, bread, pastas, sugar and starches. Glucose is a readily available fuel source for your body to use for energy, but it is not long lasting, and the process of converting carbs to glucose sends your blood sugar on a roller coaster.

Here is how it works

After consuming carbohydrate, your body begins to digest them into glucose.

This process of converting carbs to glucose causes a spike in your blood sugar and gives you a temporary energy boost (the word sugar high comes from here)

Responding to this aggressive blood sugar spike (and because the glucose in your bloodstream can be toxic), your body react by signaling to the pancreas to release the hormone insulin, which acts to remove the excess glucose from your bloodstream

The release insulin works swiftly to transport the glucose out of your bloodstream to burn as fuel and then puts the rest in storage (more on this in a minute)

As the insulin removes the glucose from your bloodstream, your blood sugar subsequently drops your energy level declines, and you feel hungry again, So the more you consume carbs, the cycle repeat itself again.

This process is why most people get hungry every minute of their lives not because of lack of their will power that causes the craving but their body is the one requesting for more carb because their blood sugar is very low.

If being on the never ending glu-coaster wasn't bad enough, I have one more important fact for you. Depending on how much energy you need (which is based primarily on your physical activity level), you burn that specific amount of glucose and the rest is stored in your body. Some of the excess is converted into glycogen and stored in your liver and muscle tissues for future use. But the remaining glucose that your body didn't use is stored as fat in the form of triglycerides. That's right; your body stores the excess glucose in your fat cells and essentially forgets about it there.

Then, of course, the whole cycles starts again. You eat more carbs at your next meal, you jump on the glu-coaster" your body uses what it needs for energy and stores the rest as fat. And those fat cells keep piling up. This is the reason you gain weight.

Another fuel source ketones, these are incredible little energy pods created by your body from stored fat. You can turn these fat cells into energy, not just any kind of energy but a long lasting and consistent energy with no afternoon crash. When you use ketone for energy, your body is using its own stored fat as fuel, thus you start losing weight.

The main purpose of ketogenic diet is to capitalize on all this by training your body to start burning ketones for energy instead of glucose. This phenomenal is called ketosis and when your body is in ketosis, it becomes a literal fat burning machine.

Ketosis

Whenever your body takes stored fat through the liver and produces ketones (small molecules used as fuel throughout the body) it is called ketosis

Why do you need to be in ketosis?

When you are in a state of ketosis, your body literally becomes a fat burning machine. Ketosis is the way for humans to operate most efficiently and can lead to numerous benefits such as weight loss, increased energy, improved focus, better sleep, clear skin, strength gain, reduce appetite, better digestion and balanced mood.

How Do You Get into Ketosis?

To get yourself into ketosis, you need to know how you consume each macronutrient daily.

There are three types of macronutrients in the human diet are they are Fats, Protein and Carbohydrate. While on ketogenic diet, your daily macronutrient breakdown should be as follows

75% healthy fats

20% quality protein

5% carbohydrates

With the above statement you will understand that 75 % of what you eat each day comes from fat as it's the most essential macronutrient that the body needs. You need fat to live. It keeps you feeling full and satisfied; prevent craving and 100 percent necessary for you to get into ketosis

Once you follow this macronutrient ratio, you can get into ketosis within two to seven days, depending on your current glycogen supply, body type and activity level. This means you can start reaping the amazing benefits of ketosis in as little as one week.

Benefits of Keto Diet

People engage themselves in keto diet because of their personal reasons, for many it's because of weight loss, while some people that don't have weight engage themselves with keto diet because of energy, clear skin or better mental focus. So before you engage yourself with ketogenic diet, ask yourself why you really want to engage yourself with this diet.

Here are some benefits of keto diet

Fat loss

If you can recall, earlier I define ketosis as a way of burning stored fat for energy. By engaging yourself with clean keto lifestyle, weight loss can often be significant and can happen quickly, because not only you are turning your body into a machine, but you are also ridding your body of processed foods, artificial ingredients and sugars that interfere with your appetite hormones

Once you are in ketosis, you seldom feel hungry, your craving subside, and you don't have to worry about counting calories. No more food drama.

Improved Brain Function

Engaging yourself with keto diet don't only helps you to lose weight but also improve cognitive function, mental clarity and to finally lift your brain fog once and for all, to cut it short, a sharper mind is most likely one of the first thing you will benefit while on ketosis.

This happens because, in comparison to glucose, ketones are actually and upgraded fuel source for your brain. Research have shown that ketones can provide as much as 70 percent of the brain's energy needs and are more energy efficient than glucose.

Fast & Sustainable Energy

Long lasting energy is one of the most important benefits of engaging yourself with keto diets. While on ketogenic diet, your energy level are stable throughout the day, meaning no mid-afternoon slumps, no insatiable craving for sugar, and no need for caffeine pick me-ups. This is because when you get off the "glu-coaster" your blood sugar levels are stabilized

Decrease Inflammation

Inflammation is always in our body. Some are advantageous like when you get a scrap, your body heals as a result of inflammation. However, chronic inflammation can become a problem

Also, when you remove processed food in your diet, you consequently eliminate all inflammation producing additives, artificial ingredients, preservatives and sweeteners, and instead fill your plate with real foods full of minerals and vitamins that work to decrease internal inflammation in your body.

How to Lose Weight with the Ketogenic Diet?

The following tips should be applied while losing weight through the ketogenic diet plan:

1. Choose a diet containing fewer carbohydrates

You need to cut down on your consumption of starch and sugar. This idea is more than a century old. There have been a lot of diet plans which are based on reducing the amount of carbs you take. The new thing with the

Ketogenic diet is that you provide your body with an alternate source of energy to depend on, which is a fat. When you do not eat carbohydrates or eat them moderately, your body is capable of burning 300 additional calories per day, even when you are resting! It means that this amount of burnt calories is equal to a gym session of moderate physical activity.

2. Eat when you feel hungry

You do not need to stay hungry all the time to lose weight. This is the most common mistake committed by people who start a low carb diet. In the Ketogenic diet, you do not have to be scared of fats.

Carbohydrates and fats are two major sources of energy for our body. If you are snatching carbs from your body, you need to give it an ample supply of fats. Low fats and low carbs equal to starvation, and we do not want that, do we? Starvation results in cravings and fatigue. That is why, people who starve give up easily on their diet plans. The better solution is to consume natural fat till the time you are satisfied. Some of the natural fats are full fat cream, butter, olive oil, meat, bacon, fatty fish, coconut oil, eggs.

3. Eat real food

This is one more common mistake made by Ketogenic followers that they get fooled by the fraudulent but creative marketing of "low carb" foods. A real Ketogenic diet should be supported by real food. It implies the food which is being eaten by humans for millions of years. For example, fish, meat, vegetables, olive oil, butter, nuts, etc.

4. Eat only If you feel hungry

You must have read tip number 2 above. In the Ketogenic diet, eat when you are hungry. Do not eat when you are not feeling hungry. Let us elaborate why we are stressing this point again. Unnecessary snacking may become a mammoth issue in the Ketogenic diet. Some products are just so easily available and they are so tempting that you cannot resist them.

5. You can skip meals

Yes, you heard it right. You can even skip breakfast if you are not feeling hungry. This holds truth for any meal.

When you are strictly following the Ketogenic diet, your hunger goes down significantly, especially if you have to lose a lot of weight. Your body is happily busy in burning excess fats and reduces your temptation to eat.

6. Wisely measure your development

Losing weight successfully might get trickier sometimes. If you focus on your weight all the time and step on the weighing scale all the time, you may get mislead. It de-motivates you and makes you anxious needlessly.

7. Be persistent

You would have all those chunks of fats around your waist and thighs in several years. So, how do you expect to lose all the extra fat in just a few weeks? If you want to shed that extra weight permanently, you have to make persistent efforts.

Foods to Avoid On Keto Diet
Fruits & Vegetables

- Apricots
- Apples
- Bananas
- Artichokes
- Beans (all varieties)
- Boysenberries
- Butternut squash
- Burdock root
- Cantaloupe
- Cherries
- Chickpeas
- Corn
- Currants
- Edamame

- Egg plants
- Dates
- Elderberries
- Gooseberries
- Grapes
- Mangoes
- Leaks
- Huckleberries
- Honeydew melons
- Kiwifruit
- Parsnips
- Peaches
- Peas
- Potatoes
- Plums
- Pineapples
- Plantains
- Prune
- Raisins

- Taro
- Turnips
- Yams
- Winter squash
- Water chestnuts

Meat and Meats Alternative

- Sausage (with fillers)
- Hot dog (with fillers)
- Seitan,
- Tofu
- Deli meat (Some not all)

Diary

- Milk
- Almond milk (sweetened)
- Coconut milk (sweetened)
- Soy milk (regular)
- Yogurt (regular)
- Nuts & Seeds
- Pistachios
- Cashew
- Chestnuts

Keto Pantry Essential

It is wise to have a well stocked pantry when you are cooking keto meals. You do not need any exotic cooking ingredients; you just need to have the basics.

Keto Cooking Staples

- Freshly ground black pepper

1. Ghee

2. Freshly ground pepper (clarified butter, without diary)

3. Olive oil

4. Grass-fed butter

In addition to these five staples, there are 10 perishable ingredients you will want to always have on hand; you just need to have the basics.

Keto Perishables

1. Avocados

2. Bacons (Uncured)

3. Eggs (pasture raised, if you can)

4. Cream cheese (Full fat, or use a diary alternative)

5. Sour cream (Full fat, or use a diary alternative)

6. Cauliflower

7. Meat (Grass fed, if you can)

8. Greens (Spinach, Kale or Arugula

9. Heavy whipping cream

10.   Garlic (Fresh or pre-minced)

Chapter Three: What is an Air Fryer?

An air fryer is a cooking appliance which helps to cook various delicious and tasty dishes at home. Those of us that make use of convection oven should expect the same experience they had with while making use of air fryer. Air fryer cooks food by circulating hot air into an air fryer chamber. This is a device where you can fry something like French fries with a little oil and that's one of the benefits of this device called Air Fryer device as it save up to 80 percent of oil while frying or cooking food. People do complain of lack of crispiness in their food, air fryer makes your food crispy you guys don't need to worry about that again.

The cooking chamber of an air fryer contains a heating element that radiates heat to cook food more appropriately and efficiently. Above the chamber is an exhaust fan that provides the required air flow, which is what allows the hot air to move around the food constantly. As a result, every part of the food is exposed to the same heating temperature. The air fryer also contains an exhaust system that keeps the temperature in check. The temperature is increased through internal pressure that produces extra air required to cook the food. Food cooked in an air fryer is healthier and contains fewer calories because it requires very little oil to produce the fried effect. Imagine being able to make crispy chips with only half a tablespoon of oil. Seems impossible? Not with an air fryer. The best part is that cooking doesn't take long. You can have crispy potatoes in just twelve minutes. Air fryers are not just better for your health; they are also good for the environment because the extra air that is produced to cook the food is filtered thoroughly before it is released, so you don't have the unpleasant odor that lingers in the kitchen whenever you fry foods the traditional way. While air fryers were originally created to air fry foods, many of the newer models now have the capability of grilling and roasting, so you can cook a variety of other foods like steaks and hamburgers.

The Benefits of Air Fryer

Less Oil and Fats

Air fryer don't require much oil to perform it magic, as it only requires a little bit oil and at the same time save 80 percent of oil during cooking. A spoon of oil is enough for air fryer to perform magic on your French fries as it makes it tender from inside and crispy outside

Time Saving

Air fryer saves a lot of time, this should be a good news to everybody most especially busy mothers because nobody want to waste his or her time preparing food the whole day.

Maintain Nutritional Values

Traditional deep-frying method destroys essential vitamins and minerals from your food. Air fryer fries your food by blowing the very hot air into a food basket. Air frying your food helps to maintain essential vitamins and nutrients into your food

So Many Cooking Options

Most of you might think that air fryer device is only meant for air frying only while you can achieve so many things like cooking, grilling and baking with your air fryer. Confuse? Nothing to be confuse about, air fryer is just like multi-cooker where you can do all type of cooking in one pot.

Less Fear of Heart-related Disease

Consuming deep-fried is not healthy to your body as it requires much oil to get your meal done. Air fryer only requires very less oil to fry your food. It also maintains essential vitamins and nutrients into your food. This device really helps to reduce heart disease.

Automatic Cooking Programs

Currently most air fryers comes with pre=programmed auto cook button. These auto cooking functions are nothing but commonly used programs like French fries, chicken fries.

All you need to do is to press the auto cook function button and your air fryer will automatically adjust the time and temperature of your air fryer.

Step-By-Step Air Frying

Like I said before, the air fryers work on the Rapid Air technology. The cooking chamber of the air fryer radiates the heat from a heating element that is close to the foods. The exhaust fan that is present above the cooking chamber, aids in the necessary airflow from the underside.

To achieve more while cooking with air fryer, here are some steps you need to follow

Prepare the Fried Foods: the first step is to prepare the foods

- To avoid sticking to the basket add a little of oil to the food and spray the base of the cooking basket mesh with some oil.
- If the food is marinated pat it dry lightly so as to prevent splattering and excess smoke. Also, empty any fat from the bottom machine.
- If using aluminum foil trim it to leave some space around the bottom basket edge.

Prior to cooking:

- Preheat the air fryer for a sufficient time until it reaches the desired temperature.

- Avoid overcrowding the food so as to leave sufficient space for air circulation.
- For premade packaged foods, ensure to reduce the conventional oven temperature by 70 degrees and lower the cook time by half.

During cook time:

- Shake the cooking basket couple of times for smaller items.
- Rotate the food item every 5-10 minutes so that cooking takes place evenly.

After cooking:

Ensure to clean the air fryer both inside and outside.

Uses of an Air Fryer

The Air Fryer is one of those appliances you can use a substitute to any other form of cooking of which includes using as oven, stovetop, and deep fryer. It comes with various handy parts and other tools that you can buy to use your Air Fryer for different cooking styles, which include the following:

Grilling

It provides the same heat to grill food ingredients without the need to flip them continuously. The hot air goes around the fryer, giving heating on all sides. The recipes include directions of how many times you ought to shake the pan during the cooking process. To make the process of grilling faster, you can use a grill pan or a grill layer. They will soak the excess fat from the meat that you are cooking to give you delicious and healthy meals.

Baking

The Air Fryer usually comes with a baking pan (or you can buy or use your own) to make treats that are typically done using an oven. You can bake goodies, such as cakes, bread, cupcakes, muffins, and brownies in your Air Fryer.

Roasting

It roasts food ingredients, which include vegetables and meat, faster than when you do it in the oven.

Frying-

This is its primary purpose, to cook fried foods with little or no oil.

Good Fats That Are Suitable for Air Frying

Most of the recipes for Air Frying require only a little oil, so non-stick oil spray is the most appropriate to use. If you want to use solid fats, melt them in the microwave first before applying them directly to the food. You have many options for healthy fats that you can use for air frying. Since you will only use a little for each food preparation, it is not ideal to stock up a lot of these oils. Store your oils in the fridge to extend the shelf life.

- ***Coconut oil*** (or coconut butter in solid form) This oil is mainly meant for Asian dishes, to make use of it, you need to leave at room temperature for ten minutes before making use of it just in case you stored it in the fridge

2. ***Almond oil*** works best as flavoring oil rather than the central cooking fat. You can brush the oil in the food ingredients five minutes before cooking. It gives a nutty taste, specifically to green veggies, such as broccoli and green beans.

3. ***Olive oil.*** It is no doubt healthy oil, but in air frying, it evaporates quickly, especially when you are cooking porous food items. These food items include eggplant, potatoes, and mushrooms, which are best prepared using oils that stay longer in the pan such as goose fat or duck fat.

4. ***Avocado oil*** .It adds a unique flavor to vegetable dishes. Store this in the fridge and leave at room temperature before using.

5. ***Sesame oil*** is not used for cooking, but only for enhancing dishes because it has a strong flavor. Don't use more than a teaspoon of this oil for every recipe.

6. ***Duck fat*** is economical since a tablespoon of this is already equal to 4 tablespoons of regular cooking oil. It stores soft in the fridge so you can use it right away.

7. **Walnut oil** is excellent flavoring oil because it gives a defined flavor to dishes, especially to risottos.

8. **Hazelnut oil**. It gives off a rich flavor to different dishes and ingredients, such as eggplant, potatoes, and risottos.

9. **Ghee** is less fattening than butter. You can use a tablespoon of ghee for recipes that require two tablespoons of butter. Store it in the fridge and leave at room temperature before using.

10. **Goose fat**. A tablespoon of this fat can do the job of up to 4 tablespoons of cooking oil. You can use ghee right out of the fridge upon opening because it remains soft.

Chapter Four: Keto Dairy Free Air Fryer Recipe
August Liver Burger

Servings: 7

Total Time: 25 Minutes

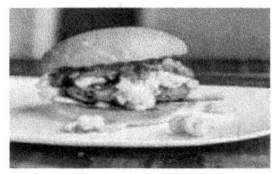

Ingredients and Quantity

½ teaspoon turmeric

½ teaspoon ground coriander

1 teaspoon ground thyme

½ teaspoon salt

2 teaspoon coconut oil

1 tablespoon almond flour

1 tablespoon coconut flour

1 teaspoon chili flakes

1-pound chicken liver

1 egg

Direction

Grin the chicken liver.

2. Put the ground chicken in the mixing bowl.

3. Beat the egg in the separate bowl and whisk it.

4. Add the turmeric, ground coriander, ground thyme, and salt in the whisked egg mixture.

5. Add the whisked egg mixture in the ground liver.

6. Next, add the coconut flour and almond flour.

7. Mix it up with the help of the spoon. You should get the non-sticky liver mixture.

8. Add more almond flour if desired.

9. Preheat the air fryer to 360 F. Then melt the coconut oil and spread the air fryer basket tray with the melted butter.

10. Make the medium liver burgers and put them in the prepared air fryer basket tray.

11. Cook the burgers for 5 minutes on each side.

12. The burger's sides should be a little bit crunchy.

13. When the liver burgers are cooked, let them chill little and then serve

Sesame Salad with Beef Strips
Servings: 5

Total Time: 22 Minutes

Ingredients and Quantity

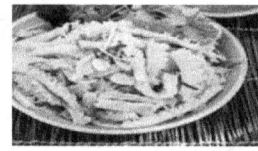

2 cup lettuce

10 oz. beef brisket

2 tablespoon sesame oil

1 tablespoon sunflower seeds

1 cucumber

1 teaspoon ground black pepper

1 teaspoon paprika

1 teaspoon Italian spices

2 teaspoon coconut oil

1 teaspoon dried dill

2 tablespoon coconut milk

Direction

Cut the beef brisket into the strips.

2. Sprinkle the beef strips with the ground black pepper, paprika, and dried dill.

3. Preheat the air fryer to 365 F.

4. Put the butter in the air fryer basket tray and melt it. Then add the beef strips and cook them for 6 minutes from 2 sides.

5. Meanwhile, tear the lettuce and toss it in the big salad bowl.

6. Crush the sunflower seeds and sprinkle the lettuce.

7. Chop the cucumber into the small cubes and add the vegetable in the salad bowl too. Then combine the sesame oil and Italian spices together.

8. Stir the oil – the dressing for the salad is cooked.

9. Sprinkle the lettuce mixture with the coconut milk and stir it using 2 wooden spatulas.

10. When the meat is cooked – let it chill until the room temperature.

11. Add the beef strips in the salad bowl.

12. Stir it gently and sprinkle the salad with the sesame oil dressing.

13. Serve the dish immediately.

Stuffed Beef Heart

Servings: 4

Total Time: 35 Minutes

Ingredients and Quantity

1-pound beef heart

1 white onion

½ cup fresh spinach

1 teaspoon salt

1 teaspoon ground black pepper

3 cups chicken stock

1 teaspoon coconut oil

Direction

Prepare the beef heart for cooking by removing all the fat from it.

2. Then peel the onion and dice it. Chop the fresh spinach.

3. Combine the diced onion, fresh spinach, and butter together. Then stir it.

4. Next, make the cut in the beef heart and fill it with the spinach-onion mixture.

5. Preheat the air fryer to 400 F and pour the chicken stock into the air fryer basket tray.

6. Then sprinkle the prepared stuffed beef heart with the salt and ground black pepper.

7. Put the prepared beef heart in the air fryer and cook it for 20 minutes.

8. When the time is over – remove the cooked heart from the air fryer and slice it

9. Then sprinkle the slices with the remaining liquid from the air fryer. Serve and enjoy!

Whole Chicken with Rosemary

Servings: 12

Total Time: 90 Minutes

Ingredients and Quantity

6-pound whole chicken

1 teaspoon kosher salt

1 teaspoon ground black pepper

1 teaspoon ground paprika

1 tablespoon minced garlic

3 tablespoon coconut oil

1 teaspoon canola oil

¼ cup water

½ white onion

Direction

1. Rub the whole chicken with the kosher salt and ground black pepper inside and outside.
2. Then sprinkle it with the ground paprika and minced garlic.
3. Peel the onion and dice it. Put the diced onion inside the whole chicken.
4. Then add the coconut oil and rub the chicken with the canola oil outside.
5. Preheat the air fryer to 360 F and pour water in the air fryer basket.
6. Then place the rack and put the whole chicken there.
7. Cook the chicken for 75 minutes.
8. When the chicken is cooked, it will have little bit crunchy skin.
9. Cut the cooked dish into the servings. Serve and enjoy

Juicy Keto Turkey Rolls

Servings: 4

Total Time: 22 Minutes

Ingredients and Quantity

1 teaspoon dried dill

1 tablespoon chives

4 teaspoon coconut oil

1-pound turkey fillet

2 tablespoon garlic clove, sliced

1 teaspoon apple cider vinegar

½ white onion

½ teaspoon salt

1 teaspoon paprika

Direction

Cut the turkey fillet into 4 parts.

2. Then beat every turkey fillet gently.

3. Sprinkle the turkey fillets with the apple cider vinegar, salt, paprika, and dried dill.

4. Chop the onion and combine it with the sliced clove.

5. Now add the chives and butter.

6. Mix the mixture until homogenous.

7. Then place the churned garlic mixture in the center of every turkey fillet.

8. Roll the fillet and secure well with toothpicks.

9. Preheat the air fryer to 360 F.

10. Put the turkey rolls in the air fryer basket tray and cook for 12 minutes.

11. Turn the rolls into another side once per coking.

12. Transfer the cooked juicy turkey rolls to the plate and serve them hot.

Keto Chicken Breast

Servings: 4

Total Time: 32 Minutes

Ingredients and Quantity

- 1 pound chicken breast, boneless, skinless
- 3 tablespoon Stevia extract
- 1 teaspoon ground white pepper
- 1/2 teaspoon paprika
- 1 teaspoon cayenne pepper
- 1 teaspoon lemongrass

- 1 teaspoon lemon zest
- 1 tablespoon apple cider vinegar
- 1 tablespoon coconut oil

Direction

1. Sprinkle the chicken breast with the apple cider vinegar.

2. Now rub the chicken breast with the ground white pepper, paprika, cayenne pepper, lemongrass and lemon zest.

3. Leave the chicken breast for 5 minutes to marinate.

4. Next, rub the chicken breast with the stevia extract and leave it for 5 minutes more.

5. Preheat the air fryer to 380 degrees F.

6. Rub the prepared chicken breast with the coconut oil and place it in the air fryer basket tray.

7. Cook the chicken for 12 minutes.

8. Turn the chicken breast into another side after 6 minutes of cooking.

- 9. Serve and enjoy hot!

Indian Lamb Meatballs

Servings: 8

Total Time: 24 Minutes

Ingredients and Quantity

- 1 garlic clove
- 1 tablespoon coconut oil
- 1 white onion
- 1/4 tablespoon turmeric
- 1/3 teaspoon cayenne pepper
- 1 teaspoon ground coriander
- 1/4 teaspoon bay leaf
- 1 teaspoon salt
  - 1 egg
- 1 teaspoon ground black pepper

Direction

1. Peel the garlic clove and mince it.

2. Combine the minced garlic with the ground lamb.

3. Now sprinkle the meat mixture with the turmeric, cayenne pepper, ground coriander, and bay leaf, salt and ground black pepper.

4. Beat the egg in the forcemeat.

5. Then grate the onion and add it in the lamb forcemeat also.

6. Mix up to make the smooth mass.

7. Preheat the air fryer to 400 degrees F.

8. Put the butter in the air fryer basket tray and melt it.

9. Then make the meatballs from the lamb mixture and place them in the air fryer basket tray.

10. Cook the dish for 14 minutes.

11. Stir the meatballs twice during the cooking.

- 12. Now serve the cooked meatballs immediately.

Pork Chops with Keto Gravy

Servings: 4

Total Time: 32 Minutes

Ingredients and Quantity

- 1 pound pork chops
- 1 teaspoon kosher salt
- 1/2 teaspoon ground cinnamon
- 1 teaspoon ground white pepper
- 1 cup heavy cream
- 6 oz. white mushrooms
- 1 tablespoon coconut oil

- 1/2 teaspoon ground ginger
- 1 teaspoon ground turmeric
- 1 white onion, chopped
- 1 garlic clove chopped

Direction

1. Sprinkle the pork chops with the kosher salt, ground cinnamon, ground white pepper and ground turmeric.

2. Preheat the air fryer to 375 degrees F.

3. Pour the heavy cream in the air fryer basket tray.

4. Then slice the white mushrooms and add them in the heavy cream.

5. Now add coconut oil, ground ginger, chopped onion and chopped garlic.

6. Cook the pork chops at 400 F for 12 minutes.

7. When the time is over stir the pork chops gently and transfers them to the serving plates. Serve and enjoy!

Keto Sandwich (Bread-Free)

Servings: 2

Total Time: 20 Minutes

Ingredients and Quantity

2 slices dairy free cheese

6 oz. ground chicken

1 teaspoon tomato puree

1 teaspoon cayenne pepper

- 1 egg

½ teaspoon salt

1 tablespoon dried dill

½ teaspoon olive oil

2 lettuce leaves

Direction

Combine the ground chicken with the cayenne pepper and salt.

2. Add the dried dill and stir it.

3. Then beat the egg in the ground chicken mixture and stir it well with the help of the spoon.

4. After this, make 2 medium burgers from the ground chicken mixture.

5. Preheat the air fryer to 380 F.

6. Spray the air fryer basket tray with the olive oil and place the ground chicken burgers there.

7. Cook the chicken burgers for 10 minutes.

8. Next, transfer the cooked chicken burgers in the lettuce leaves.

9. Sprinkle them with the tomato puree and cover with the dairy free cheese slices and serve!

Winter Squash Tots

Servings: 5

Total Time: 25 Minutes

Ingredients and Quantity

- 1 cup pumpkin puree
- 1 tablespoon almond flour
- 1/2 teaspoon almond flour
- 1/4 teaspoon salt
- 1/4 cup coconut flour
- 1 teaspoon olive oil
- 1/4 teaspoon turmeric

Direction

1. Take the big bowl and combine the pumpkin puree, almond flour, ground nutmeg, salt and turmeric.

2. Mix the mixture with the help of a fork.

3. Then add the coconut flour.

4. Mix it up again. The pumpkin mixture should be non-sticky.

5. Separate the pumpkin dough into 5 parts and form 5 tots.

6. Preheat the air fryer to 360 degrees F.

7. Spray the air fryer with the olive oil inside and cook the pumpkin tots for 10 minutes.

- 8. Serve chill and enjoy!

Spiced Cucumber Chips

Servings: 5

Total Time: 21 Minutes

Ingredients and Quantity

- 1 pound cucumber
- 1 teaspoon salt
- 1 tablespoon smoked paprika
- 1/2 teaspoon garlic powder

Direction

1. Wash the cucumbers carefully and slice them into chips shape.

2. Sprinkle the sliced cucumber chips with the salt, smoked paprika and garlic powder.

3. Preheat the air fryer to 370 degrees F.

4. Place the cucumber chips for 11 minutes.

5. Then transfer the cucumber chips in the paper towel and chill them well.

6. Serve the cucumber chips immediately.

Bacon Omelet

Servings: 6

Total Time: 23 Minutes

Ingredients and Quantity

6 eggs

¼ cup almond milk

½ teaspoon turmeric

½ teaspoon salt

1 tablespoon dried dill

4 oz. bacon

1 teaspoon coconut oil

Direction

Beat the egg in the mixer bowl and add almond milk.

2. Mix up the mixture with the help of the mixer until it is smooth.

3. Add the turmeric, salt, and dried dill. Then slice the bacon.

4. Preheat the air fryer to 360 F and put the sliced bacon in the air fryer basket tray.

5. Cook the bacon for 5 minutes.

6. Next, turn the bacon into another side and pour the egg mixture over it.

7. Cook the omelet for 8 minutes more.

8. Next, transfer it to the plate and slice into the servings. Serve and enjoy!

Keto Fish Fries

Servings: 6

Total Time: 16 Minutes

Ingredients and Quantity

- 1 pound cod fillet
- 2 large eggs
- 1 tablespoon coconut oil
- 1/2 teaspoon salt or to taste
- 1 teaspoon ground black pepper

- 1 teaspoon turmeric
- 1 teaspoon paprika

Direction

1. Cut the cod fillet into 6 parts, of fry's size.

2. Beat the egg in the bowl and whisk it.

3. Add the salt, ground black pepper, turmeric and paprika and stir.

4. Now dip the cod fillets in the egg mixture.

5. Preheat the air fryer to 360 degrees F.

6. Spray the cod fillets with the coconut oil and put them in the air fryer rack.

7. Cook the dish for 6 minutes.

8. Stir the cod fries after 4 minutes of cooking.

9. Remove the cooked fish fries from the air fryer.

10. Serve the dish with keto sauce.

Mushroom Omelet

Servings: 9

Total Time: 22 Minutes

Ingredients and Quantity

1 tablespoon flax seeds

7 eggs

½ cup dairy free cream cheese

4 oz. white mushrooms

1 teaspoon olive oil

1 teaspoon ground black pepper

½ teaspoon paprika

¼ teaspoon salt

Direction

Slice the mushrooms and sprinkle them with the salt, paprika, and ground black pepper.

2. Preheat the air fryer to 400 F.

3. Spray the air fryer basket tray with olive oil inside and place the sliced mushrooms there.

4. Cook the mushrooms for 3 minutes.

5. Stir them carefully after 2 minutes of cooking.

6. Meanwhile, beat the eggs in the bowl. Add the cream cheese and flax seeds.

7. Mix the egg mixture up carefully until you get the smooth texture.

8. Then pour the omelet mixture into the air fryer basket tray over the mushrooms.

9. Stir the omelet gently and cook it for 7 minutes more.

10. Next, remove the cooked omelet from the air fryer basket tray using the wooden spatula.

11. Slice it into the servings and serve!

Shredded Beef with Herbs

Servings: 8

Total Time: 37 Minutes

Ingredients and Quantity

1 teaspoon thyme

1 teaspoon ground black pepper

1 garlic clove, peeled

3 tablespoon coconut oil

1 bay leaf

1 teaspoon salt

1 teaspoon dried dill

1 teaspoon mustard, low carb, sugar free

4 cup chicken stock

2-pound beef steak

Direction

Preheat the air fryer to 360 F.

2. Meanwhile, combine the thyme, ground black pepper, salt, dried dill, and mustard in the small mixing bowl.

3. After this, sprinkle the beefsteak with the spice mixture from the both sides.

4. Massage the beefsteak with the help of the fingertip to make the meat soak the spices.

5. Then pour the chicken stock in the air fryer.

6. Add the prepared beef steak and bay leaf.

7. Cook the beefsteak for 20 minutes.

8. When the time is over, strain the chicken stock and discard the beefsteak from the air fryer.

9. Shred the meat with the help of 2 forks and return it back in the air fryer basket tray.

10. Add butter and cook the meat for 2 minutes at 365 F.

11. After this, mix the shredded meat carefully with the help of the fork.

12. Transfer the dish to the serving bowls.

Beef Strips with Zucchini Spirals

Servings: 8

Total Time: 28 Minutes

Ingredients and Quantity

1-pound beef brisket

1 teaspoon ground black pepper

1 tomato

1 teaspoon salt

1 zucchini

1 teaspoon olive oil

1 teaspoon Italian spices

4 tablespoon water

Direction

Cut the beef brisket into the strips.

2. Sprinkle the beef strips with the ground black pepper and salt.

3. Next, chop the tomato roughly and transfer it to the blender.

4. Blend it well until you get the smooth puree.

5. Now spray the air fryer basket tray with the olive oil inside and put the beef strips there.

6. Cook the beef strips for 9 minutes at 365 degrees F.

7. Stir the beef strips carefully after 4 minutes of cooking.

8. Meanwhile, wash the zucchini carefully and make the spirals from the vegetable with the help of the spiralizer.

9. When the time of the cooking of the meat is finished, add the zucchini spirals over the meat.

10.   Then sprinkle it with the tomato puree, water, and Italian spices.

11.   Cook the dish for 4 minutes more at 360 F.

12.   When the time is over and the dish is cooked, stir it gently with the help of the wooden spatula.

13.   Serve the dish immediately.

Chapter Five: Keto Air Fryer Weight Loss Recipes

Keto Chinese Greens

Servings: 2

Total Time: 20 Minutes

Ingredients and Quantity

- 1 tablespoon chives
- 1 teaspoon sesame seeds
- 1 tablespoon apple cider vinegar
- 2 tablespoon coconut butter
- 1 tablespoon canola oil
- 1/2 teaspoon salt
- 8 oz. bok choy
- 1 tablespoon garlic, sliced
- 1/2 teaspoon stevia extract

Direction

1. Preheat the air fryer to 360 degrees F.

2. Slice the bok choy and place it in the air fryer basket tray.

3. Now sprinkle the sliced bok choy with the salt and coconut butter.

4. Cook the bok choy for 10 minutes.

5. When the bok choy is cooked, allow it to cool.

6. Then transfer to the serving plate.

7. Combine the chives, sesame seeds, apple cider vinegar, canola oil and stevia extract in the shallow bowl.

8. Add the sliced garlic and mix it.

9. Now sprinkle the cooked bok choy with the prepared garlic mixture.

10. Stir gently.

11. Serve and enjoy!

Turnip Mash

Servings: 6

Total Time: 24 Minutes

Ingredients and Quantity

- 5 turnip
- 3 oz. coconut butter

- 1/2 white onion, grated
- 1 teaspoon salt
- 1 cup coconut cream

Direction

1. Preheat the air fryer to 400 degrees F.

2. Peel the turnip and chop them.

3. Place the chopped turnips in the air fryer basket tray.

4. Add coconut butter, grated onion, and salt and coconut cream.

5. Cook the dish for 14 minutes.

6. Allow the cooked turnip to chill for 5 minutes when the time has elapsed.

7. Now use the hand blender to blend the turnip mixture into the mash.

8. Serve the cooked turnip mash warm.

Air Fryer Creamy Snow Peas

Servings: 4

Total Time: 12 Minutes

Ingredients and Quantity

- 1/2 cup coconut cream

- 1 teaspoon coconut butter
- 1 teaspoon salt
- 1 teaspoon paprika
- 1 pound snow peas
- 1/4 teaspoon nutmeg

Direction

1. Preheat the air fryer to 400 degrees F.

2. Wash the snow peas carefully and place them in the air fryer basket tray.

3. Now sprinkle the snow peas with the butter, salt, paprika, nutmeg and heavy cream.

4. Cook the snow peas for 5 minutes.

5. When the time has elapsed, shake the snow peas gently and transfer them to the serving plate.

6. Serve and enjoy!

Keto Summer Vegetables

Servings: 4

Total Time: 30 Minutes

Ingredients and Quantity

- 1 eggplant
- 1 tomato

- 1 zucchini
- 1 white onion
- 2 green peppers
- 1 teaspoon paprika
- 1 tablespoon canola oil
- 1/2 teaspoon ground nutmeg
- 1/2 teaspoon ground thyme
- 1 teaspoon salt

Direction

1. Preheat the air fryer to 390 degrees F.

2. Wash the eggplant, tomato and zucchini carefully.

3. Peel the onion and chop all the prepared vegetable roughly.

4. Now place the chopped vegetable in the air fryer basket tray.

5. Sprinkle the vegetables with the paprika, canola oil, ground nutmeg, ground thyme and salt.

6. Stir the vegetables carefully with the help of 2 spatulas.

7. Cut the green peppers into squares.

8. Add the pepper squares into the vegetable mixture and stir gently.

9. Cook the dish for 15 minutes.

10. stir the vegetables after 10 minutes.

11. Allow them to chill for 4 minutes when the cooking time has elapsed.

- 12. Serve and enjoy!

Liver Pate

Servings: 7

Total Time: 20 Minutes

Ingredients and Quantity

1-pound chicken liver

1 teaspoon salt

4 tablespoon coconut butter

1 cup water

1 teaspoon ground black pepper

1 onion

½ teaspoon dried cilantro

Direction

Chop the chicken liver roughly and place it in the air fryer basket tray.

2. Then peel the onion and dice it.

3. Pour the water in the air fryer basket tray and add the diced onion.

4. Preheat the air fryer to 360 F and cook the chicken liver for 10 minutes.

5. When the time is over, strain the chicken liver mixture to discard it from the liquid.

6. Transfer the chicken liver mixture into the blender.

7. Add the coconut butter, ground black pepper, and dried cilantro.

8. Blend the mixture till you get the pate texture.

9. Then transfer the liver pate in the bowl and serve it immediately or keep in the fridge. Serve!

Flax Meal Porridge

Servings: 4

Total Time: 13 Minutes

Ingredients and Quantity

2 tablespoon sesame seeds

4 tablespoon chia seeds

1 cup almond milk

3 tablespoon flax meal

1 teaspoon stevia

1 tablespoon coconut butter

½ teaspoon vanilla extract

Direction

Preheat the air fryer to 375 F.

2. Put the sesame seeds, chia seeds, almond milk, flax meal, stevia, and coconut butter in the air fryer basket tray.

3. Add the vanilla extract and cook the porridge doe 8 minutes.

4. After that, stir the porridge carefully and leave it for 5 minutes to rest.

5. Then transfer the meal into the serving bowls or ramekins and serve!

Keto-Jerk Chicken Wings

Servings: 4

Total Time: 29 Minutes

Ingredients and Quantity

- 1 pound chicken wings

- 1/2 teaspoon salt

- 1 tablespoon garlic powder
- 1/4 teaspoon ground black pepper
- 1/4 teaspoon cayenne pepper
- 1/2 teaspoon ground ginger
- 1 tablespoon mustard, low carb
- 1 tablespoon tomato puree

Direction

1. Place the chicken wings in the mixing bowl.

2. Sprinkle the chicken wings with the salt, garlic powder, ground black pepper, cayenne pepper, ground ginger and mustard.

3. Mix the chicken wings carefully.

4. Then add the tomato puree and mix the chicken wings carefully again.

5. Let the chicken wings for 10 minutes to marinate.

6. Preheat the air fryer to 370 degrees F.

7. Place the chicken wings in the air fryer basket tray and cook the dish for 14 minutes.

8. When the chicken wings are cooked, transfer them to the serving plate.

- 9. Serve and enjoy!

Toasted Nuts

Servings: 4

Total Time: 14 Minutes

Ingredients and Quantity

- 1/4 cup hazelnuts
- 1/4 cup walnuts
- 1/2 cup pecans
- 1/2 macadamia nuts
- 1 tablespoon olive oil
- Salt to taste

Direction

1. Preheat the air fryer to 320 degrees F.

2. Place the hazelnuts, walnuts, pecans and macadamia nuts in the air fryer.

3. Cook the nuts for 8 minutes.

4. Now stir the nuts after 4 minutes of the cooking.

5. Next, sprinkle the nuts with olive oil and salt and shake them well.

6. Cook the nuts for another 1 minute.

7. Then transfer the cooked nuts to the serving bowls.

- 8. Serve and enjoy!

Keto Nuggets

Servings: 5

Total Time: 25 Minutes

Ingredients and Quantity

- 1 pound chicken fillet
- 1/2 teaspoon salt or to taste
- 1/2 teaspoon ground black pepper
- 1/2 teaspoon chili pepper
  - 2 eggs
- 1/2 cup coconut flour

Direction

1. Cut the chicken fillet into the nugget size pieces.

2. Crack the eggs into the bowl and beat them.

3. Combine the coconut flour, chili pepper, salt and ground black pepper in the big mixing bowl.

4. Shake it well to make the mixture homogenous

5. Dip the nuggets in the beaten egg.

6. Then coat the chicken nuggets in the almond flour mixture.

7. Preheat the air fryer to 360 degrees F.

8. Transfer the coated chicken nuggets in the air fryer rack and cook them for 10 minutes.

- 9. Serve hot and enjoy!

Eggplant Chips

Servings: 10

Total Time: 28 Minutes

Ingredients and Quantity

- 1 teaspoon onion powder
- 1 teaspoon salt
- 3 big eggplants
- 1 teaspoon paprika
- 1/2 teaspoon ground black pepper
- 1 tablespoon canola oil

Direction

1. Wash the eggplants and slice them into chips shapes.

2. Sprinkle the eggplant slices with the salt to help make the eggplant less juicy and bitter.

3. Then dry the eggplant slices and sprinkle them with the onion powder, paprika and ground black pepper.

4. Stir the eggplant slices with the help of your fingertips.

5. Now preheat the air fryer to 400 degrees F.

6. Place the eggplant slices in the air fryer rack and cook them for 13 minutes.

7. The temperature of the cooking may vary a little depending on the thickness of the eggplant slices.

8. When the chips are cooked, cool them to room temperature.

- 9. Serve and enjoy!

Winter Squash Tots

Servings: 5

Total Time: 25 Minutes

Ingredients and Quantity

- 1 cup pumpkin puree
- 1 tablespoon almond flour
- 1/2 teaspoon almond flour
- 1/4 teaspoon salt

- 1/4 cup coconut flour
- 1 teaspoon olive oil
- 1/4 teaspoon turmeric

Direction

1. Take the big bowl and combine the pumpkin puree, almond flour, ground nutmeg, salt and turmeric.

2. Mix the mixture with the help of a fork.

3. Then add the coconut flour.

4. Mix it up again. The pumpkin mixture should be non-sticky.

5. Separate the pumpkin dough into 5 parts and form 5 tots.

6. Preheat the air fryer to 360 degrees F.

7. Spray the air fryer with the olive oil inside and cook the pumpkin tots for 10 minutes.

- 8. Serve chill and enjoy!

Spiced Cucumber Chips

Servings: 5

Total Time: 21 Minutes

Ingredients and Quantity

- 1 pound cucumber

- 1 teaspoon salt
- 1 tablespoon smoked paprika
- 1/2 teaspoon garlic powder

Direction

7. Wash the cucumbers carefully and slice them into chips shape.

8. Sprinkle the sliced cucumber chips with the salt, smoked paprika and garlic powder.

9. Preheat the air fryer to 370 degrees F.

10. Place the cucumber chips for 11 minutes.

11. Then transfer the cucumber chips in the paper towel and chill them well.

- 12. Serve the cucumber chips immediately.

Beef Strips with Zucchini Spirals

Servings: 8

Total Time: 28 Minutes

Ingredients and Quantity

1-pound beef brisket

1 teaspoon ground black pepper

1 tomato

1 teaspoon salt

1 zucchini

1 teaspoon olive oil

1 teaspoon Italian spices

4 tablespoon water

Direction

14. Cut the beef brisket into the strips.

15. Sprinkle the beef strips with the ground black pepper and salt.

16. Next, chop the tomato roughly and transfer it to the blender.

17. Blend it well until you get the smooth puree.

18. Now spray the air fryer basket tray with the olive oil inside and put the beef strips there.

19. Cook the beef strips for 9 minutes at 365 degrees F.

20. Stir the beef strips carefully after 4 minutes of cooking.

21. Meanwhile, wash the zucchini carefully and make the spirals from the vegetable with the help of the spiralizer.

22. When the time of the cooking of the meat is finished, add the zucchini spirals over the meat.

23. Then sprinkle it with the tomato puree, water, and Italian spices.

24. Cook the dish for 4 minutes more at 360 F.

25. When the time is over and the dish is cooked, stir it gently with the help of the wooden spatula.

26. Serve the dish immediately.

Stuffed Beef Heart

Servings: 4

Total Time: 35 Minutes

Ingredients and Quantity

1-pound beef heart

1 white onion

½ cup fresh spinach

1 teaspoon salt

1 teaspoon ground black pepper

3 cups chicken stock

1 teaspoon coconut oil

Direction

10. Prepare the beef heart for cooking by removing all the fat from it.

11. Then peel the onion and dice it. Chop the fresh spinach.

12. Combine the diced onion, fresh spinach, and butter together. Then stir it.

13. Next, make the cut in the beef heart and fill it with the spinach-onion mixture.

14. Preheat the air fryer to 400 F and pour the chicken stock into the air fryer basket tray.

15. Then sprinkle the prepared stuffed beef heart with the salt and ground black pepper.

16. Put the prepared beef heart in the air fryer and cook it for 20 minutes.

17. When the time is over – remove the cooked heart from the air fryer and slice it

18. Then sprinkle the slices with the remaining liquid from the air fryer. Serve and enjoy!

Whole Chicken with Rosemary

Servings: 12

Total Time: 90 Minutes

Ingredients and Quantity

6-pound whole chicken

1 teaspoon kosher salt

1 teaspoon ground black pepper

1 teaspoon ground paprika

1 tablespoon minced garlic

3 tablespoon coconut oil

1 teaspoon canola oil

¼ cup water

½ white onion

Direction

1. Rub the whole chicken with the kosher salt and ground black pepper inside and outside.
2. Then sprinkle it with the ground paprika and minced garlic.
3. Peel the onion and dice it. Put the diced onion inside the whole chicken.
4. Then add the coconut oil and rub the chicken with the canola oil outside.
5. Preheat the air fryer to 360 F and pour water in the air fryer basket.
6. Then place the rack and put the whole chicken there.
7. Cook the chicken for 75 minutes.
8. When the chicken is cooked, it will have little bit crunchy skin.
9. Cut the cooked dish into the servings. Serve and enjoy!

Juicy Keto Turkey Rolls

Servings: 4

Total Time: 22 Minutes

Ingredients and Quantity

1 teaspoon dried dill

1 tablespoon chives

4 teaspoon coconut oil

1-pound turkey fillet

2 tablespoon garlic clove, sliced

1 teaspoon apple cider vinegar

½ white onion

½ teaspoon salt

1 teaspoon paprika

Direction

Cut the turkey fillet into 4 parts.

2. Then beat every turkey fillet gently.

3. Sprinkle the turkey fillets with the apple cider vinegar, salt, paprika, and dried dill.

4. Chop the onion and combine it with the sliced clove.

5. Now add the chives and butter.

6. Mix the mixture until homogenous.

7. Then place the churned garlic mixture in the center of every turkey fillet.

8. Roll the fillet and secure well with toothpicks.

9. Preheat the air fryer to 360 F.

10. Put the turkey rolls in the air fryer basket tray and cook for 12 minutes.

11. Turn the rolls into another side once per coking.

12. Transfer the cooked juicy turkey rolls to the plate and serve them hot.

Swedish Meatballs

Servings: 6

Total Time: 26 Minutes

Ingredients and Quantity

- 1 tablespoon almond flour
- 1 pound ground beef
- 1 teaspoon dried parsley
- 1 teaspoon dried dill
- 1/2 teaspoon ground nutmeg
- 1 oz. white onion, chopped
- 1 teaspoon garlic powder
- 1 teaspoon salt
- 1/2 cup heavy cream
- 1/4 cup chicken stock
- 1 teaspoon mustard

- 1 teaspoon ground black pepper
- 1 tablespoon butter

Direction

1. Combine the ground beef and almond flour together in the bowl.

2. Add the dried dill, dried parsley, ground nutmeg, garlic powder, chopped onion, salt, ground black pepper and mustard.

3. Mix the mixture up to get the smooth forcemeat.

4. Now make the meatballs from the beef forcemeat.

5. Preheat the air fryer to 380 degrees F.

6. Put the beef meatballs in the air fryer basket tray.

7. Add the butter and cook the dish for 5 minutes.

8. After this, turn the meatballs into another side.

9. Sprinkle the meatballs with the heavy cream and chicken stock.

10. Cook the meatballs for 6 minutes more.

11. When the meatballs are cooked, serve them immediately with the cream gravy.

- 12. Serve and enjoy!

Turmeric Cauliflower Rice

Servings: 6

Total Time: 18 Minutes

Ingredients and Quantity

- 1 white onion, diced
- 3 tablespoon coconut butter
- 1 teaspoon salt
- 1 pound cauliflower
- 1 teaspoon turmeric
- 1 teaspoon minced garlic
- 1 teaspoon ground ginger
- 1 cup chicken stock

Direction

1. Wash the cauliflower and chop it roughly.

2. Then place the chopped cauliflower in the blender and blend it till you get the rice texture of the cauliflower.

3. Transfer the cauliflower rice to the mixing bowl.

4. Add the diced onion.

5. Next, sprinkle the vegetable mixture with the salt, turmeric, minced garlic and ground ginger and mix everything up.

6. Preheat the air fryer to 370 degrees F.

7. Put the cauliflower rice mixture there.

8. Add the coconut butter and chicken stock.

9. Cook the cauliflower rice for 10 minutes.

10. When the time is over, remove the cauliflower rice from the air fryer and strain the excess liquid.

- 11. Stir gently. Serve and enjoy!

Spiced Asparagus

Servings: 6

Total Time: 15 Minutes

Ingredients and Quantity

- 1 pound asparagus
- 1 teaspoon salt
- 1 teaspoon chili flakes
- 1/2 teaspoon ground white pepper
- 1 tablespoon sesame oil
- 1 tablespoon flax seeds

Direction

1. Combine the sesame oil with the salt, chili flakes and ground white pepper.

2. Churn the mixture.

3. Preheat the air fryer to 400 degrees F.

4. Place the asparagus in the air fryer basket tray and sprinkle it with the sesame oil-spiced mixture.

5. Cook the asparagus for 6 minutes.

6. When the dish is cooked, allow it to chill for a while.

- 7. Then serve and enjoy!

Sriracha Broccoli

Servings: 5

Total Time: 16 Minutes

Ingredients and Quantity

- 1 teaspoon sriracha
- 1 tablespoon canola oil
- 1 tablespoon flax seeds
- 1 teaspoon kosher salt
- 1 pound broccoli
- 4 tablespoons chicken stock

Direction

1. Wash the broccoli and separate it into the florets.

2. Now combine the chicken stock, ground white pepper, flax seeds and sriracha.

3. Add the canola oil and whisk the mixture.

4. Preheat the air fryer to 400 degrees F.

5. Put the broccoli florets in the air fryer basket rack and sprinkle the vegetables with the sriracha mixture.

6. Cook the broccoli for 6 minutes.

7. When the time is over, shake the broccoli gently and transfer it to the serving plates.

- 8. Serve and enjoy!

Blackberry Muffins

Servings: 5

Total Time: 25 Minutes

Ingredients and Quantity

1 teaspoon apple cider vinegar

1 cup almond flour

4 tablespoon coconut butter

6 tablespoon almond milk

1 teaspoon baking soda

3 oz. blackberry

½ teaspoon salt

3 teaspoon stevia

1 teaspoon vanilla extract

Direction

Put the almond flour in the mixing bowl.

2. Add the baking soda, salt, stevia, and vanilla extract.

3. After this, add coconut butter, almond milk, and apple cider vinegar.

4. Smash the blackberries gently and add them to the almond flour mixture.

5. Stir it carefully with the help of the fork until the mass is homogeneous.

6. After this, leave the muffin mixture for 5 minutes in warm place.

7. Meanwhile, preheat the air fryer to 400 F.

8. Prepare the muffin forms. Then pour the dough in the muffin forms.

9. Fill only ½ part of every muffin form.

10. When the air fryer is preheated – put the muffing forms with the filling in the air fryer basket.

11. Close the air fryer. Cook the muffins for 10 minutes.

12. When the time is over – remove the muffins from the air fryer basket.

13. Chill them until they are warm. Serve!

Egg Soufflé

Servings: 2

Total Time: 16 Minutes

Ingredients and Quantity

2 eggs

2 tablespoon coconut cream

1 tablespoon dried parsley

¼ teaspoon ground chili pepper

¼ teaspoon salt

Direction

Preheat the air fryer to 391 F.

2. Meanwhile, crack the eggs into the bowl and add the heavy cream.

3. Whisk the mixture carefully until you get the smooth liquid texture.

4. After this, sprinkle the egg mixture with the dried parsley, ground chili pepper, and salt.

5. Mix it up with the help of the spoon. Then take 2 ramekins and pour the soufflé mixture there.

6. Place the ramekins in the air fryer basket and cook for 8 minutes.

7. When the time is over and the soufflé is cooked, remove the ramekins from the air fryer basket and chill for 2-3 minutes.

8. Serve the dish and enjoy!

Wrapped Bacon Asparagus

Servings: 6

Total Time: 25 Minutes

Ingredients and Quantity

- 7 oz. bacon, sliced
- 14 oz. asparagus
- 1 teaspoon salt
- 1 teaspoon ground black pepper
- 1 teaspoon sesame oil
- 1 teaspoon paprika

Direction

1. Wrap the asparagus in the sliced bacon.

2. Preheat the air fryer to 380 F.

3. Put the wrapped asparagus in the air fryer and sprinkle the vegetables with the salt, ground black pepper, paprika and sesame oil.

4. Cook the asparagus for 5 minutes.

5. After this, turn the asparagus to another side and cook it for 5 minutes more.

6. Cook the broccoli for 6 minutes.

7. When the time is over, shake the broccoli gently and transfer It to the serving plates.

- 8. Serve and enjoy

Buffalo Cauliflower

Servings: 5

Total Time: 25 Minutes

Ingredients and Quantity

8 oz. cauliflower

6 tablespoon almond flour

1 teaspoon chili pepper

teaspoon ground black pepper

1 tomato

1 teaspoon minced garlic

½ teaspoon salt

1 teaspoon olive oil

Direction

Wash the cauliflower carefully and separate it into the medium florets.

2. Sprinkle the cauliflower florets with the salt.

3. Next, chop the tomato roughly and transfer it to the blender.

4. Blend it well. Then add the chili pepper, cayenne pepper, ground black pepper, and minced garlic.

5. Blend the mixture. Then preheat the air fryer to 350 F.

6. Sprinkle the air fryer basket with the olive oil inside.

7. Sprinkle the cauliflower florets with the blended tomato mixture generously.

8. Now coat the cauliflower florets in the almond flour.

9. Place the coated cauliflower florets in the air fryer basket and cook the dish for 15 minutes.

10. Shake the cauliflower florets every 4 minutes.

11. When the cauliflower is cooked – it will have light brown color.

12. Transfer it to the serving plates and serve!

Hemp Seeds Porridge

Servings: 3

Total Time: 25 Minutes

Ingredients and Quantity

2 tablespoon flax seeds

4 tablespoon hemp seeds

1 tablespoon coconut butter

¼ teaspoon salt

1 teaspoon stevia

7 tablespoon almond milk

½ teaspoon ground ginger

Direction

Place the flax seeds and hemp seeds in the air fryer basket.

2. Sprinkle the seeds with the salt and ground ginger.

3. Combine the almond milk and stevia together.

4. Stir the liquid and pour it in the seeds mixture.

5. Now add coconut butter.

6. Preheat the air fryer to 370 F and cook the hemp seeds porridge for 15 minutes.

7. Stir it carefully after 10 minutes of cooking.

8. When the time is over, remove the hem porridge from the air fryer basket tray and chill it for 3 minutes.

9. Transfer the Hemp Seeds porridge in the serving bowls.

Parsley Coconut Butter Mushrooms

Servings: 5

Total Time: 17 Minutes

Ingredients and Quantity

- 10 oz. white mushrooms

- 1 white onion, sliced
- 1 teaspoon olive oil
- 1/3 teaspoon garlic powder
- 3 tablespoon coconut butter
- 1/2 cup coconut cream
- 2 tablespoon dried parsley
- 1/2 teaspoon salt

Direction

1. Slice the white mushrooms and sprinkle them with the garlic powder and salt.

2. Preheat the air fryer to 400 degrees F.

3. Put the sliced mushrooms in the air fryer basket tray.

4. Sprinkle the mushrooms with the olive oil and then add the onion.

5. Cook the mushrooms for 2 minutes.

6. Now stir the sliced mushrooms gently.

7. Add the coconut butter and cream.

8. Sprinkle the mushrooms with the dried parsley.

9. Stir the mushrooms carefully again and cook them for additional 5 minutes.

- 10. When the time has elapsed, stir the dish very well. Serve and enjoy!

Keto Crab Mushrooms

Servings: 5

Total Time: 20 Minutes

Ingredients and Quantity

- 7 oz. crab meat
- 10 oz. white mushrooms
- 1/2 teaspoon salt
- 1/4 cup fish stock
- 1 teaspoon coconut butter
- 1/4 teaspoon ground coriander
- 1 teaspoon dried cilantro
- 1 teaspoon butter

Direction

1. Chop the crab meat and sprinkle it with the salt and dried cilantro.

2. Mix the crab meat carefully.

3. Now preheat the air fryer to 400 degrees F.

4. Chop the white mushrooms and combine them with the crab meat.

5. Next, add the fish stock, ground coriander and butter.

6. Transfer the side dish mixture in the air fryer basket tray.

7. Stir gently with the help of the plastic spatula.

8. Cook the side dish for 5 minutes.

9. When the time has elapsed, allow the dish to cool for about 5 minutes.

- 10. Serve and enjoy!

Bacon Cabbage

Servings: 5

Total Time: 25 Minutes

Ingredients and Quantity

- 4 oz. bacon, chopped
- 10 oz. white cabbage, shredded
- 1/4 white onion, diced
- 1/2 teaspoon salt
- 1 teaspoon paprika
- 1 teaspoon butter

- 1/2 teaspoon ground black pepper

Direction

1. Preheat the air fryer to 360 degrees F.

2. Put the chopped bacon in the air fryer basket tray.

3. Sprinkle it with salt and paprika.

4. Now add coconut butter and cook the bacon for 8 minutes.

5. Next, add the shredded cabbage, diced onion, butter and ground black pepper.

6. Stir the mixture carefully and cook it for 7 more minutes.

7. The cabbage will be soft when the time has elapsed.

8. Stir the side dish carefully.

- 9. Serve hot and enjoy!

Garlic Zucchini Pate

Servings: 4

Total Time: 27 Minutes

Ingredients and Quantity

- 2 garlic cloves, chopped
- 1 tablespoon coconut butter
- 1 teaspoon salt

- 1/2 teaspoon ground black pepper
- 2 zucchini
- 1/2 tablespoon olive oil

Direction

1. Peel the zucchini and grate it.

2. Now combine the grated zucchini with the salt and ground pepper and stir the zucchini.

3. Preheat the air fryer to 390 degrees F.

4. Put the grated zucchini in the air fryer basket tray.

5. Add olive oil and chopped garlic clove and cook it for 8 minutes.

6. Next, stir the zucchini carefully and add butter.

7. Cook the zucchini pate for 4 minutes more at 400 degrees F.

8. The zucchini pate will be smooth and soft when the time has elapsed. Remove it from the air fryer and allow it to cool to room temperature.

- 9. Serve and enjoy!

Chapter Six: Air Fryer Gluten-Free Recipes
Onion Rings

Serve: 4

Prep: 10 min Cook: 15-20 min

Ingredients and Quantity

- 1 cup Rice Flour
- 1 cup Gluten-free all purpose flour
- ¼ tsp Salt
- ¼ tsp Pepper
- 1 tsp Paprika
- 1 tsp Baking soda
- 1 tsp Garlic powder
- 1 ½ cups Club soda (chilled)
- 2 Onions (chopped into rings)
- 2 cups Buttermilk

Directions:

- Put the onion rings in the buttermilk and refrigerate for an hour. Combine all the dry ingredients in a bowl.

2. Pick up the onion rings from the buttermilk and then dip into the club soda.

3. Dredge it with the flour-spice mixture.

4. Air fry for 15-20 minutes until ready.

5. Serve and enjoy

Crispy Tofu

Serve: 2

Prep: 10 min Cook: 18 min

Ingredients and Quantity

- 1 (8oz) package Firm tofu (rinsed, cubed)
- 2 tbsp Nutritional yeast
- 1 tbsp Brown rice flour
- 2 tbsp Soy sauce
- 1 tsp Sesame oil
- 1 tsp Water
- ½ tsp Garlic powder

Directions:

- Mix together all the dry ingredients in a bowl. Gradually mix in the wet ingredients, stirring well.

2. Marinate the tofu in the mixture for ½ hour.

3. Sprinkle a little rice flour over the marinated tofu cubes.

4. Air fry for 18 minutes at 350 degrees Fahrenheit.

5. Serve and enjoy

Mushroom & risotto chorizo balls

Serve: 2-4

Prep: 10 min Cook: 20 min

Ingredients and Quantity

- 1 serving No stir mushroom risotto
- 3.5 oz GF Breadcrumbs
- 3.5 oz GF chorizo (sliced)
- ½ cup GF Plain flour
- ¼ cup Milk

Directions:

- Prepare the no-stir mushroom risotto adding the chorizo at the time of adding the mushrooms.

2. Place the risotto in the refrigerator to cool.

3. Roll the risotto mixture into balls, roll them into the flour, then dip them into the egg and finally dredge them in breadcrumbs.

4. Preheat the air fryer to 392 degrees Fahrenheit.

5. Place the balls in the air fryer in a single layer and cook for 20 minutes.

Orange Sesame Chicken

Serve: 3

Prep: 10 min Cook: 20 min

Ingredients and Quantity

- ¼ cup Chicken: Sesame seeds
- 1 cup Rice Krispies cereal (crushed)
- 1 ½ cup Rice flour
- 1 Eggs (beaten)
- 2 Egg Yolks (beaten)
- 1 tbsp Sesame oil
- 17 ½ oz Chicken thighs (skinless, boneless, cubed)
- Salt to taste Orange

Sauce

- ¼ cup Rice vinegar
- ½ cup Water
- ½ cup Orange Marmalade (shred-less)
- 1 cup Brown sugar
- 1 cup Orange juice
- 3 tbsp GF soy sauce
- 1 Garlic clove
- 1 tsp Ginger (grated)
- 3 tbsp Cornstarch
- Orange zest of ½ orange

Directions:

- Combine the rice Krispies cereal, salt and sesame seeds in a bowl.

2. Dredge the chicken first in flour, then coat with the beaten eggs and then dredge it in the cereal mixture.

3. Place the chicken in the air fryer and drizzle the sesame oil over the chicken.

4. Add more sesame oil up to the air fryer max oil line. Cook for 20 minutes.

5. Combine all the sauce ingredients in a saucepan apart from the cornstarch and bring to boil.

6. Mix together a little sauce with the cornstarch and add it back to the saucepan.

7. Toss the chicken in the sauce and sprinkle the sesame seeds onto it.

8. Serve and enjoy

Banana Chips

Serve: 4

Prep: 10 min Cook: 20 min

Ingredients and Quantity

- 2 Raw green bananas (washed, sliced)

- 1 tsp Turmeric powder
- Salt to taste
- 1 cup Water

Directions:

- Mix together the water salt and turmeric, stirring until dissolved.

2. Place the banana slices in the turmeric water for 15 minutes.

3. Drain, dry and spread as a single layer on the air fryer basket. Bake for 12-14 minutes at 392 degrees Fahrenheit tossing it midway and spraying with some non-stick oil.

4. Serve and enjoy

Egg & Potato Breakfast Platter

Serve: 2

Prep: 10 min Cook: 25 min

Ingredients and Quantity

- Eggs
- ½ cup Heavy cream
- 1 tbsp Sunflower oil
- 3 Eggs
- Salt and pepper to taste

Potatoes:

- 1 tbsp Sunflower oil
- 1 tbsp Onion powder
- 1 tablespoon Paprika
- 1 tablespoon Garlic powder
- 3 Potatoes (peeled, cubed)
- Salt and pepper to taste

Directions:

- Toss together the potatoes, onion powder; garlic powder and paprika in the air fryer pan, drizzling some oil over them. Cook for 20 minutes.

2. Transfer onto a platter and season with salt and pepper.

3. Scramble the egg, cream and salt together in a bowl.

4. Heat oil in the air fryer pan and add the eggs to it. Cook for 4 minutes and transfer to the platter.

5. Season with salt and pepper.

6. Serve and enjoy

Cheesy Bacon Quiche

Serve: 2

Prep: 10 min Cook: 32 min

Ingredients and Quantity

- ½ cup Bisquick Gluten-free mix
- ¼ cup Bacon (cooked, crumbled)
- ¼ cup Cheddar cheese (shredded)
- 2 Eggs
- 2 tbsp Shortening
- 1 cup Whipping cream
- Salt and pepper to taste

Directions:

- Mix together the Bisquick and shortening in a bowl until well mixed.

2. Add a tablespoon of water and using your hand kneads into dough.

3. Place the dough in a quiche pan and gently press it on the base and half inch up the sides.

4. Place in the air fryer basket and cook for 10 minutes at 400 degrees Fahrenheit.

5. Layer the bacon and the cheese over the crust. Beat together the eggs, salt, pepper and whipping cream and pour it over the cheese layer.

6. Place in the air fryer and cook for 22 minutes at 360 degrees Fahrenheit.

7. Serve and enjoy

Karaage Chicken

Serve: 2

Prep: 10 min Cook: 17 min

Ingredients and Quantity

- 15 ¾ oz Chicken thigh (2 cm pieces)
- 1 cup Potato starch
- 2 tbsp Marinade: Sake
- 4 tbsp Organic soy sauce
- 1 tbsp Ground ginger
- 3 tsp Raw sugar
- 4 tsp Olive oil
- 2 Garlic cloves (minced)

Directions:

- Mix together all the marinade ingredients and marinate the chicken with it for 4 hours in the refrigerator.

2. Coat the chicken with the potato starch and place in the air fryer preheated to 320 degrees Fahrenheit for 5 minutes.

3. Cook at 392 degrees Fahrenheit for 12 minutes, flipping the pieces midway.

4. Serve and enjoy

Crisped Calamari

Serve: 2

Prep: 5 min Cook: 8 min

Ingredients and Quantity

- 1 cup GF oats
- 1 Egg (beaten)
- 1 Lemon (juice & rind)
- 1 tbsp Paprika
- 1 tsp Parsley
- Salt and pepper to taste
- 1 oz Calamari (sliced into rings)

Directions:

- Blend the oats in a blender to make crumbs. Combine the oat crumbs with the rest of the seasonings.

2. Season the calamari with salt, pepper and lemon.

3. Dredge the calamari rings with crumb mixture and place in an air fryer preheated to 360 degrees Fahrenheit.

4. Cook for 8 minute and serve

Choco-Banana Cake

Serve: 10

Prep: 10 min Cook: 35 min

Ingredients and Quantity

- 10 Bananas
- 10 tsp Organic cocoa powder
- 4 tbsp Honey
- 8 Eggs
- 1 Avocado

Directions:

- Combine all the ingredients except the avocado in a blender and blend until smooth. Leave aside a little for the icing layer and the rest you divide between two baking pans.

2. Cook for 35 minutes in an air fryer preheated to 360 degrees Fahrenheit.

3. Remove from the tins and leave to cool on a wire rack. In the batter kept aside, mix in the avocado.

4. Spread the avocado mixture on one of the cake and place the other cake over.

5. Leave to refrigerate until the icing sets.

6. Serve and enjoy once set

Crispy Garlic

Serve: 4

Prep: 10 min Cook: 35 min

Ingredients and Quantity

- 16 pieces Chicken wings (rinsed, dried)
- ¾ cup Potato Starch
- ¼ cup Honey
- ¼ cup Butter
- ½ tsp Kosher salt
- 4 tbsp Garlic (minced)

Directions:

- Coat the chicken wings with potato starch and place in the air fryer for 25 minutes at 380 degrees Fahrenheit, tossing the wings every 5 minutes.

2. Cook for 10 minutes at 400 degrees Fahrenheit. Simultaneously, melt the butter in a saucepan over

medium flame and mix in the garlic, cooking for 5 minutes.

3. Mix in the salt and honey and simmer for 20 minutes on low flame, stirring often.

4. Pour the sauce over the chicken.

5. Serve and enjoy

Shrimps with Spicy Orange Marmalade

Serve: 2

Prep: 10 min Cook: 20 min

Ingredients and Quantity

- 8 Shrimps (shelled, deveined)
- 8 oz Coconut milk
- ½ cup Coconut (shredded, sweetened)
- ½ cup Panko bread
- ½ tsp Cayenne pepper
- ¼ tsp Kosher salt
- ½ cup Orange Marmalade
- ¼ tsp Ground pepper
- 1 tbsp Honey
- 1 tsp Mustard
- ¼ tsp Hot sauce

Directions:

- Whisk the coconut milk in a bowl, seasoning it with salt and pepper. Mix the coconut, cayenne pepper, salt, black pepper and panko in another bowl.

2. Dip the shrimps first in the coconut milk and then dredge with the coconut mixture.

3. Place in an air fryer and cook at 350 degrees Fahrenheit for 20 minutes.

4. Whisk together the hot sauce, mustard, honey and marmalade in a bowl.

5. Serve the shrimps with the sauce.

Turkey Meatballs

Serve: 8

Prep: 10 min Cook: 10 min

Ingredients and Quantity

- 2 packages Ground turkey
- 1 cup Crushed chips
- 1 tbsp Onion flakes
- 2 Garlic cloves
- 2 Eggs
- 1 tbsp Montreal steak spice
- 1 tbsp Roasted garlic seasoning

Directions:

- Combine the spices, chips, salt and pepper in a bowl, missing well.

2. Marinate the meat with the garlic and egg and then mix in the spiced chip mix. Shape into meatballs.

3. Spray the air fryer basket preheated for 3 minutes, with a non-stick spray.

4. Place the meatballs in it and cook for 10 minutes.

Buffalo Meat balls

Serve: 4

Prep: 10 min Cook: 14 min

Ingredients and Quantity

- 1 lb Ground buffalo
- 2 tbsp Tomato paste
- 1 tbsp Garlic powder
- 1 tbsp Onion powder
- 2 tsp Basil
- Salt and pepper to taste

Directions:

- Combine the meat with the rest of the ingredients in a bowl and mix well. Shape into meatballs.

2. Place the meatballs in the air fryer and cook for 14 minutes at 360 degrees Fahrenheit.

3. Serve and enjoy

Chicken Nuggets

Serve: 1

Prep: 10 min Cook: 20 min

Ingredients and Quantity

- 4 oz Ground chicken
- 2 tbsp Golden flax meal
- 1 tsp Coconut flour
- Ground spices as per choice

Directions:

- Mix together all the ingredients except the chicken in a bowl. Shape the chicken portions into nuggets.

2. Coat the nuggets with the flax mixture and place in a baking sheet lined with parchment paper.

3. Place in the air fryer and cook for 20 minutes at 375 degrees Fahrenheit.

4. Serve and enjoy

Almond Flavored Chicken Nuggets

Serve: 1

Prep: 10 min Cook: 20 min

Ingredients and Quantity

- 4 oz Ground chicken
- 2 tbsp Almond flour
- Ground spices as per choice

Directions:

- Mix together all the ingredients except the chicken in a bowl. Shape the chicken portions into nuggets.

2. Coat the nuggets with the almond mixture and place in a baking sheet lined with parchment paper.

3. Place in the air fryer and cook for 20 minutes at 375 degrees Fahrenheit.

4. Serve and enjoy

Crispy Polenta

Serve: 1

Prep: 10 min Cook: 12 min

Ingredients and Quantity

- ¼ tube Polenta (chopped into 4 wedges and then slice)
- 2 tsp Nutritional yeast

- ½ tsp Smoked paprika
- 1/8 tsp Salt

Directions

- Preheat the air fryer to 400 degrees Fahrenheit.

2. Shake together the rest of the ingredients in a Ziploc bag.

3. Add the polenta and shake again.

4. Place in the air fryer and cook for 10-12 minutes, tossing once in between.

5. Serve and enjoy

Roasted Pork Ribs

Serve: 2

Prep: 5 min Cook: 35 min

Ingredients and Quantity

- 1 rack Ribs
- 1 tbsp Olive oil
- 1 tbsp Herb mixture
- 2 tbsp Black pepper sauce

Directions:

- Marinate the ribs with the rest of the ingredients overnight in a refrigerator.

2. Preheat the air fryer to 320 degrees Fahrenheit. Place the ribs in the air fryer and cook for 30 minutes.

3. Increase the temperature to 392 degrees Fahrenheit and cook for another 5 minutes covered with aluminum foil.

4. Serve and enjoy

Sweet & Sour Pork

Serve: 4

Prep: 10 min Cook: 20 min

Ingredients and Quantity

- ½ oz Pork (cubed)

Marinade:

- 1 tsp Light soy sauce
- 2 tsp Maggi seasoning
- 1 tsp Sesame oil
- 1 tsp Black pepper

Sauce

- 1 Onion (sliced)
- 1 Fresh pineapple slice (cubed)
- 1 tbsp Garlic (minced)
- 1 tbsp Worcestershire sauce
- 1 Egg
- Flour as required
- Sugar to taste
- 2 tbsp Oyster sauce
- 2 tbsp Tomato sauce

Directions:

- Preheat the air fryer to 320 degrees Fahrenheit. Dip the pork in egg and then dredge with flour.

2. Cook in the air fryer for 20 minutes.

3. For the sauce, heat a little oil in a saucepan and sauté the garlic and onions in it.

4. Mix in the rest of the sauce ingredients, stirring well.

5. Add the pork, mixing to coat with the sauce.

6. Serve and enjoy

Baked Crayfish

Serve: 3

Prep: 5 min Cook: 20 min

Ingredients and Quantity

- 17 ½ oz Crayfish (washed & scrubbed)
- 1 tsp Salted butter (diced) - (2 inch x 1cm) block Garlic
- Salt and pepper to taste
- 3 Cream cubes

Directions:

- Preheat the air fryer to 360 degrees Fahrenheit for 5 minutes.

2. Place the crayfish on an aluminum foil, bottom-side upwards.

3. Spread the cream cubes and butter over the fish and season it with salt, garlic and pepper.

4. Fold the foil to make a parcel and place in the air fryer basket.

5. Cook in the air fryer for 20 minutes at 375 degrees Fahrenheit.

6. Serve and enjoy

Garlic Butter Clams

Serves: 4

Prep: 5 min Cook: 15 min

Ingredients and Quantity

- 35 oz Clams (washed, scrubbed)
- 2 tsp Salted butter (diced) - (2 inch x 1cm) block Garlic (diced)
- 2 tsp Ginger (diced)
- Salt and pepper to taste
- Rice wine to taste

Directions:

- Preheat the air fryer to 392 degrees Fahrenheit for 5 minutes.

2. Place the clams on an aluminum foil, bottom-side upwards.

3. Spread the garlic, ginger and butter over the clams and season it with salt and pepper. Pour over the wine.

4. Fold the foil to make a parcel and place in the air fryer basket.

5. Cook in the air fryer for 14-15 minutes. If any clams remain unopened, discard them.

Tuna Cutlets

Serve: 4

Prep: 10 min Cook: 7 min

Ingredients and Quantity

- 1 can Tuna (in brine, drained)
- 1 Egg
- ½ can Champignon mushrooms (chopped)
- Salt and pepper to taste

Directions:

- Preheat the air fryer to 360 degrees Fahrenheit for 5 minutes.

2. Combine all the ingredients in a bowl and mix well.

3. Shape into cutlets and place in the air fryer. Cook for 7 minutes.

4. Serve and enjoy

Cheesy Spicy Paneer Patties

Serve: 4

Prep: 10 min Cook: 10 min

Ingredients and Quantity

- 2 cups Paneer (grated)
- 1 cup Pizza cheese (grated)
- ½ tsp Garlic powder
- ½ tsp Chaat masala
- 1 Onion (chopped)
- ½ tsp Salt
- ½ tsp Oregano seasoning
- 1 tsp Butter

Directions:

- Combine all the ingredients in a bowl and mix well. Shape into cutlets and place in the air fryer.

2. Cook for 10 minutes at 360 degrees Fahrenheit.

3. Serve and enjoy

Quinoa Broccoli Fritters

Serve: 3

Prep: 10 min Cook: 20 min

Ingredients and Quantity

- 1 cup Broccoli (separated into florets)
- 1 cup Quinoa (cooked)
- ½ cup Parmesan cheese
- 2 Eggs (whisked)
- 1 tsp Olive oil (for drizzling)

Directions:

- Combine all the ingredients in a bowl and mix well.

2. Take a tablespoon of the mixture for each fritter and place on a baking paper in your air fryer. Drizzle a little oil on top.

3. Cook for 10 minutes at 360 degrees Fahrenheit on one side.

4. Flip and cook for another 10 minutes.

5. Serve and enjoy

Lamb Meatballs

Serve: 4

Prep: 10 min Cook: 15 min

Ingredients and Quantity

- 8 ¾ oz Lamb meat (ground)
- 2 tbsp Mint (chopped)
- 5 ¼ oz Haloumi (grated)
- 1 Egg (whisked)
- 1 tsp Olive oil (for drizzling)

Directions:

- Combine all the ingredients in a bowl and mix well. Roll portions of the mixture into meatballs and place on a baking paper in your air fryer.

2. Drizzle a little oil on top. Cook for 15 minutes at 392 degrees Fahrenheit rolling the balls mid-way through.

3. Serve and enjoy

Fish & Chips

Serve: 2

Prep: 10 min Cook: 10 min

Ingredients and Quantity

- 10 ½ oz Haddock Fish Filet (quartered)
- 10 ½ oz Potatoes (chopped into chips)
- 2 Eggs (beaten)
- 2 tbsp Vegetable oil
- ½ tbsp Lemon juice
- 2 oz Tortilla chips (crumbed)
- 1 tsp Mint sauce
- 1 tsp Butter
- Salt and pepper to taste

Directions:

- Preheat the air fryer to 360 degrees Fahrenheit. Season the fish with salt, pepper and lemon juice.

2. Dip the fish in egg and then dredge in the tortilla crumbs.

3. Place the fish and the chips in the air fryer. Cook for 15 minutes.

4. Increase the temperature to 392 degrees Fahrenheit and cook for another 5 minutes.

5. Serve and enjoy

Cheese Straws

Serve: 8

Prep: 10 min Cook: 20 min

Ingredients and Quantity

- 1 Cauliflower (separated into florets)
- 1 Egg
- 3.5 oz GF oats (crumbed)
- 1 Onion (peeled, diced)
- 5 ½ oz Cheddar cheese
- 1 tsp Mixed herbs
- 1 tsp Mustard
- Salt and pepper to taste

Directions:

- Steams the cauliflower for 20 minutes and leaves to cool, squeezing the excess moisture.

2. Combine half the cauliflower in a bowl with the rest of the ingredients and mix well, adding in the rest of the cauliflower gradually.

3. Twist the mixture into strips of straw and place in the air fryer at 360 degrees Fahrenheit.

4. Cook for 10 minutes on either side.

5. Serve and enjoy

Crisped Broccoli

Serve: 2

Prep: 45 min Cook: 10 min

Ingredients and Quantity

- 17 ½ oz Broccoli (separated into florets)
- 1 tbsp Chickpea flour
- 2 tbsp Marinade: Yoghurt
- ¼ tsp Turmeric powder
- ½ tsp Salt
- ½ tsp Red chili powder
- ¼ tsp Chaat masala

Directions:

- Soak the broccoli in water with 2 teaspoon salt for ½ hour. Drain and wipe.

2. Combine all the marinade ingredients in a bowl and mix well.

3. Toss in the broccoli and marinate for 15 minutes covered in the refrigerator.

4. Preheat the air fryer to 392 degrees Fahrenheit. Place the broccoli in the air fryer basket.

5. Cook for 10 minutes shaking the basket midway.

6. Serve and enjoy

Chicken Wings

Serve: 4

Prep: 15 min Cook: 25 min

Ingredients and Quantity

- 1 cup Glutinous rice flour
- 1 Egg (beaten)
- 1 lb Chicken wings (cut)
- 2 tsp Cajun seasoning

Directions:

1. Coat the chicken wings in some flour.

2. Dip the chicken wings in the egg and coat with the rest of the flour.

3. Refrigerate for a couple of hours and then place in the air fryer. Cook for 25-30 minutes.

4. Season with the seasoning, toss and serve.

Potato–Plantain Kebabs

Serve: 4

Prep: 10 min Cook: 18 min

Ingredients and Quantity

- 2 Plantains (unpeeled, sliced)
- 4 Potatoes
- 1 Onion (chopped finely)
- Salt to taste
- Red chili powder to taste
- 1 tbsp Ginger-garlic paste
- 3 tbsp Chickpea flour
- ½ tsp Garam masala
- 1 tbsp Tandoori masala
- Oil for brushing
- 2 tbsp Coriander leaves

Directions:

- Place the plantains and potatoes in a pressure pan along with water. Peel the potatoes and plantains.

2. Mash the plantains and potatoes and mix in the rest of the ingredients.

3. Preheat the air fryer to 360 degrees Fahrenheit for 10 minutes and brush the basket with oil.

4. Shape the mixture into kebabs and place into the air fryer.

5. Air fry for 18 minutes, flipping and brushing the kebabs with oil.

6. Serve and enjoy

Tandoori Chicken

Serve: 4

Prep: 15 min Cook: 30 min

Ingredients and Quantity

- 4 Chicken legs (With Thigh)
- 3 tsp Ginger paste
- 3 tsp Garlic paste
- Salt to taste
- 3 tbsp Lemon juice
- 2 tbsp Tandoori masala powder
- 1 tsp Roasted cumin powder
- 1 tsp Garam masala powder
- 2 tsp Red chili powder
- 1 tsp Turmeric powder
- 4 tbsp Hung curd
- Orange food color a pinch
- 2 tsp Kasuri Methi
- 1 tsp Black pepper powder

- 2 tsp Coriander powder

Directions:

- Marinate the chicken with the rest of the ingredients and leave refrigerated covered for 12 hours.

2. Line the air fryer basket with foil and preheat it to 440 degrees Fahrenheit.

3. Air fry for 18 minutes, tossing midway.

4. Serve and enjoy once done

Chapter Seven: Air Fryer Vegan Recipes
Turmeric Potato Chips

Serve: 2

Prep: 5 min Cook: 15 min

Ingredients and Quantity

- 5 Potatoes (chopped into chips)
- 1 tsp Turmeric powder
- 2 tsp Olive oil
- Salt and pepper to taste

Sauce:

- ¼ cup Sunflower seeds
- ¼ tsp Turmeric powder
- ½ tsp Fresh turmeric
- ¼ cup Water
- 1 Garlic clove
- Lemon juice of 1 lemon

Directions:

- Toss the chips with the rest of the chips ingredients and place in the air fryer at 360 degrees Fahrenheit for 15-20 minutes.

2. Blend all the sauce ingredients in a high-speed blender.

3. Serve the chips with the sauce.

Spinach Potato Kebabs

Serve: 2

Prep: 10 min Cook: 20 min

Ingredients and Quantity

- 2 Potatoes (peeled, boiled, mashed)
- 1 cup Spinach (blanched, chopped finely)
- 1 cup Green peas
- 1 tbsp Flaxseed powder
- 1 Green chili (chopped finely)
- 1 tbsp Gram flour
- 1 tsp Cumin powder
- ½ tsp Garam masala
- Salt to taste
- Oil for brushing

Directions:

- Preheat the air fryer to 392 degrees Fahrenheit for 5 minutes. Microwave the peas for 5 minutes.

2. Combine all the ingredients apart from the oil and mix well.

3. Shape into kebabs and place in the air fryer basket. Cook for 10 minutes.

4. Brush with oil, flip the kebabs and cook for another 10 minutes.

5. Serve and enjoy

Avocado Fries

Serve: 3-4

Prep: 10 min Cook: 10 min

Ingredients and Quantity

- 1 Haas avocado (peeled, pitted, sliced)
- ½ tsp Salt
- ½ cup Panko breadcrumbs
- Aquafaba of 1 (15 oz) white bean can

Directions:

- Mix together the salt and breadcrumbs in a bowl. Dip the avocado slices in the aquafaba and then dredge it with the breadcrumbs.

2. Place in the air fryer basket in a single layer.

3. Cook for 10 minutes at 390 degrees Fahrenheit, shaking the basket midway.

4. Serve and enjoy

Apple Chips

Serve: 2

Prep: 5 min Cook: 7-8 min

Ingredients and Quantity

- 1 Apple (peeled, cored, sliced thinly)
- Salt just a pinch
- 1 tbsp Sugar
- ¼ tsp Ground cinnamon

Directions:

- Preheat the air fryer to 390 degrees Fahrenheit. Place the apple in the air fryer basket and sprinkle a mixture of the rest of the ingredients over it.

2. Cook for 7-8 minutes flipping the slices midway.

3. Serve and enjoy

Rice Stuffed Tomatoes

Serve: 4

Prep: 10 min Cook: 22 min

Ingredients and Quantity

- 4 Tomatoes
- 1 Stuffing: Garlic clove (crushed)
- ½ tbsp Oil
- 1 tbsp Soy sauce
- 2 cups Cooked rice (cooled)
- 1 Carrot (diced)
- 1 cup Frozen peas
- 1 Onion (diced)

Directions:

- Preheat the air fryer to 360 degrees Fahrenheit. Chop the tops off the tomatoes, discarding the seeds.

2. For the stuffing, heat oil in a skillet and sauté the onion, garlic, peas and carrots in it for 2-3 minutes.

3. Mix in the soy sauce and the rice. Stuff the tomatoes with the rice mixture.

4. Air fry for 20 minutes and serve immediately

Breakfast Burritos

Serve: 2

Prep: 10 min Cook: 8-10 min

Ingredients and Quantity

- 2 tbsp Cashew butter
- 2 tbsp Tamari
- 1 tbsp Liquid smoke

- 1 tbsp Water
- 4 pieces Rice paper (hydrated)
- 2 servings Vegan egg scramble
- 1/3 cup Sweet potato cubes (roasted)
- 8 strips Red pepper (roasted)
- 1 Broccoli (sautéed)
- 6 stalks Fresh asparagus
- Kale Handful

Stuffing:

- 1 Garlic clove (crushed)
- ½ tsp Oil
- 1 tbsp Soy sauce
- 2 cups Cooked rice (cooled)
- 1 Carrot (diced)
- 1 cup Frozen peas
- 1 Onion (diced)

Directions:

- Preheat the air fryer to 350 degrees Fahrenheit. Whisk together the tamari, cashew butter, water and liquid smoke.

2. Add the rest of the ingredients into the rice papers, distributing equally, fold and roll.

3. Dip the rolls in the tamari mixture and place on a baking sheet.

4. Place in the air fryer and cook for 8-10 minutes.

5. Serve and enjoy

Cauliflower Fried Rice

Serve: 8

Prep: 20 min Cook: 40 min

Ingredients and Quantity

- 1 tbsp Sesame oil
- 1 tbsp Peanut oil
- 1 tbsp Soy sauce
- 4 Garlic cloves (minced)
- 1 tbsp Ginger (minced)
- ½ Lemon (juiced)
- 1 Cauliflower (chopped into florets)
- 1 can Water chestnuts (drained, chopped)
- ¾ cup Peas
- 2 cans Mushrooms (drained)
- ½ cup Egg substitute

Directions:

- Place the cauliflower in a blender and blend until you get a rice consistency.

2. Combine the oils, lemon juice, soy sauce, ginger, chestnuts, cauliflower rice and garlic in the air fryer bowl.

3. Cook for 20 minutes and then add the peas and mushrooms. Cook for another 15 minutes.

4. Cook the egg substitute in a pan with a little oil to make an omelet. Chop it up.

5. Add to the fried rice and cook for another 5 minutes.

6. Serve once done

Fish Taco Wraps

Serve: 4

Prep: 10 min Cook: 15 min

Ingredients and Quantity

- 4 Burrito size tortillas
- 1 Onion (peeled, diced)
- 1 Red bell pepper (cored, seeded, diced)
- 2 cobs Fresh grilled corn
- 4 pieces Fishless filet
- ½ cup Mango salsa
- 4 tbsp Shredded vegan cheese
- Mixed greens (radicchio, romaine, spinach)
- Tortilla chips

Directions:

- Preheat the air fryer to 400 degrees Fahrenheit. Sauté the bell pepper and onions in a pan over medium flame for 5 minutes.

2. Add the corn and stir cook for another 2 minutes.

3. Cook the fishless filets in the air fryer for 6 minutes and then chop into pieces.

4. Spoon the corn mix into the tortillas and place a few fishless filet pieces over it along with some salsa.

5. Sprinkle some tortilla chips and greens and wrap the tortillas.

6. Air fry the wraps for 6 minutes at 350 degrees Fahrenheit.

7. Serve and enjoy

Vegan Balls

Serve: 6 servings

Prep: 20 min Cook: 20 min

Ingredients and Quantity

- 7 oz Cauliflower
- 3 ½ oz Sweet potato
- 2 oz Carrot
- 3 oz Parsnips
- 2 tsp Garlic puree
- 1 tsp Chives
- 1 tsp Paprika
- 1 tsp Mixed spice
- 2 tsp Oregano

- ½ cup Desiccated coconut
- 1 cup GF Oats
- Salt and pepper to taste

Directions:

- Combine the veggies in a food processor and process until it becomes breadcrumbs. Squeeze to discard the excess moisture.

2. Transfer into a bowl and mix in the rest of the ingredients. Shape into balls and refrigerate for 2 hours.

3. Place in the air fryer, cooking for 10 minutes at 320 degrees Fahrenheit and then roll around.

4. Cook for another 10 minutes at 392 degrees Fahrenheit.

5. Serve and enjoy

Sweet Potato Popcorn

Serve: 4

Prep: 10 min Cook: 40 min

Ingredients and Quantity

- 5 oz Sweet Potatoes (peeled, diced)
- 4 tbsp Coconut milk
- 1 Spring onion (diced)
- 1 White onion (peeled, diced)

- 1 tsp Garlic puree
- 1 tsp Ginger puree
- 1 tsp Chives
- Salt and pepper to taste

Directions:

- Preheat the air fryer to 360 degrees Fahrenheit. Steam the sweet potatoes for around 20 minutes.

2. Leave to cool and then mash them. Add the rest of the ingredients and mix well.

3. Roll into small balls and place in a baking sheet lined with parchment paper. Cook for 20 minutes.

4. Serve with barbeque sauce.

Stuffed Bell Pepper

Serve 6

Prep: 10 min Cook: 10 min

Ingredients and Quantity

- 6 Bell peppers (tops chopped, seeds and pith removed)
- 1 Carrot (diced)
- 1 Onion (diced)
- 1 Potato (diced)

- 1 Vegan bread roll (diced)
- 2 Garlic cloves (diced finely)
- ½ cup Peas
- 2 tsp Herb mix
- 1/3 cup Vegan cheese (grated)

Directions:

- Preheat the air fryer to 360 degrees Fahrenheit. Combine all the ingredients except the bell pepper and grated cheese in a bowl and mix well.

2. Stuff the mixture into the bell peppers. Cook in the air fryer for 5 minutes.

3. Sprinkle the grated cheese on top and cook for more 5 minutes.

4. Serve and enjoy

Spiced Peanuts

Serve: 3

Prep: 5 min Cook: 7 min

Ingredients and Quantity

- 1 cup Raw peanuts
- 1 tsp Red chili powder
- 1 tsp Salt
- ½ tsp Dry mango powder
- 2 tsp Cooking oil

Directions:

- Preheat the air fryer to 320 degrees Fahrenheit for 5 minutes.

2. Toss together the peanuts, oil and salt. Air fry for 7 minutes

3. Sprinkle the mango powder and red chili powder.

4. Serve and enjoy

Khichdi Balls

Serve: 4

Prep: 10 min Cook: 30 min

Ingredients and Quantity

- ½ cup Split brown chickpeas
- ½ cup Rice
- 1 Tomato
- 2 Onions
- 1 Bell pepper
- ¼ oz Cumin
- 2 Green chilies
- ½ tbsp Red chili powder
- Salt to taste

Directions:

- Cook the khichdi with the chickpeas and rice and leave to cool.

2. Add in the rest of the ingredients and mix well.

3. Shape into small balls and then cook in a preheated air fryer for 10-12 minutes at 360 degrees Fahrenheit.

4. Serve and enjoy

Chickpea Samosa

Serve: 4

Prep: 15 min Cook: 15 min

Ingredients and Quantity

Dough:

- 1 cup Whole wheat flour
- 1 tbsp Oil
- ½ tsp Carom seeds
- Water as required
- Salt to taste

Filling:

- 1 Onion (chopped finely)
- ½ tsp Ginger paste
- 1 cup Black chickpeas (boiled)
- 1 tsp Mango powder
- ½ tsp Garam masala
- 1 tsp Cumin powder

- 1 Green chili (chopped finely)
- Oil for brushing
- Salt to taste

Directions:

- Combine all the dough ingredients in a bowl and knead it to form dough.

2. Heat a pan and sauté the ginger and onions in it. Mix in the chickpeas and spices, cooking until the mixture dries up. Leave aside.

3. Roll portions of the dough into rounds, chopping the rounds into half.

4. Twist the rounds into a cone, place some filling at the center and seal it up using some water.

5. Preheat the air fryer to 392 degrees Fahrenheit. Air fry the samosas for 7 minutes.

6. Brush them with oil, flip them and cook for another 6 minutes.

7. Serve and enjoy

Sago Carrot Cutlets

Serve: 4

Prep: 5 min Cook: 10 min

Ingredients and Quantity

- 17 ½ oz Potatoes (boiled)
- 2 pieces Bread slices (moist, cut into pieces)
- 1 cup Sago (soaked)
- 1 cup Carrot (grated)
- Salt to taste
- Dry mango powder to taste
- Red chili powder to taste
- ½ tsp Ajwain
- 2 tsp Groundnuts (crushed)

Directions:

- Combine all the ingredients in a bowl and mix well. Shape into cutlets. Preheat the air fryer to 360 degrees Fahrenheit.

2. Place the cutlets in the air fryer and brush some oil over it. Cook for 10 minutes.

3. Serve and enjoy

Corn Vadas

Serve: 2

Prep: 5 min Cook: 10 min

Ingredients and Quantity

- ½ cup Split brown chickpeas
- 2 tbsp American corn
- ½ tsp Ginger garlic paste
- 1 Fresh bread slice (crumbed)

- 2 Green chilies
- Salt to taste
- Cooking soda a pinch
- 1 tsp Oil

Directions:

- Blend together the green chilies, chickpeas and corn to make a coarse paste.

2. Transfer into a bowl and mix in the rest of the ingredients. Shape into cutlets.

3. Preheat the air fryer to 360 degrees Fahrenheit for 5 minutes. Cook the vadas in the air fryer for 8 minutes.

4. Serve and enjoy

Lemon Flavored Green Beans

Serve: 4

Prep: 5 min Cook: 10 min

Ingredients and Quantity

- 1 lb Green beans (de-stemmed)
- 1 Lemon (juiced)
- Salt and pepper to taste
- ¼ tsp Oil

Directions:

- Toss together all the ingredients. Cook in the air fryer for 10-12 minutes at 400 degrees Fahrenheit.

2. Serve once done

Crispy Spanish Potatoes

Serve: 3

Prep: 10 min Cook: 35 min

Ingredients and Quantity

- 1 ½ lbs Small red potatoes (quartered, boiled until just tender)
- 1 tbsp Water
- Salt to taste
- 1 tsp Tomato paste
- ½ tbsp Brown rice flour
- 1 tsp Smoked Spanish paprika
- 1 tsp Hot smoked paprika
- ½ tsp Garlic powder
- ½ tsp Salt

Directions:

- Mix together the tomato paste and water in a bowl. Mix together the flour with the rest of the ingredients except the potatoes.

2. Toss together the potatoes with the tomato paste mix and the flour mix.

3. Preheat the air fryer for 3 minutes at 360 degrees Fahrenheit. Cook the potatoes for 12-20 minutes in the air fryer shaking the basket once midway.

4. Serve once done

Baked Tofu Fingers

Serve: 2-4

Prep: 10 min Cook: 25 min

Ingredients and Quantity

- 14 oz Firm tofu (cut into strips)
- ¼ cup Japanese panko breadcrumbs
- 2 tsp Onion powder
- 2 tsp Garlic powder
- 1 tbsp Dried Basil
- 1 tbsp Dried oregano
- 1 tsp Ground black pepper
- ½ tsp Salt
- 2 tsp Canola oil (for frying)
- ¼ cup Soy milk
- 4 tbsp Nutritional yeast

Directions:

- Heat oil in a pan and sauté the breadcrumbs, onion powder, garlic powder, basil, oregano, salt, pepper, for 2 minutes.

2. Dip the tofu first in soy milk and coat with nutritional yeast, finally dredging it in the breadcrumbs.

3. Preheat the air fryer for 3 minutes at 340 degrees Fahrenheit. Cook the tofu for 20 minutes in the air fryer flipping once midway.

4. Serve and enjoy

Crispy Kale

Serve: 2-4

Prep: 10 min Cook: 10 min

Ingredients and Quantity

- 1 bunch Tuscan Kale (ribs & stems removed; leaves cut)
- 2 tbsp Olive oil
- ½ tsp Kosher salt
- ¼ tsp Ground black pepper

Directions:

- Toss together all the ingredients in a bowl.

2. Place in the air fryer basket in batches cooking for 5 minutes, tossing the chips midway.

3. Serve and enjoy

Chapter Eight: Air Fryer Low-Carb Recipes
Cheesy Paneer Patties

Serve: 4

Prep: 10 min Cook: 10 min

Ingredients and Quantity

- 2 cups Paneer (grated)
- 1 cup Pizza cheese (grated)
- ½ tsp Garlic powder
- ½ tsp Chaat masala
- 1 Onion (chopped)
- ½ tsp Salt
- ½ tsp Oregano seasoning
- 1 tsp Butter

Directions:

- Combine all the ingredients in a bowl and mix well. Shape into cutlets and place in the air fryer.
2. Cook for 10 minutes at 360 degrees Fahrenheit.
3. Serve and enjoy

Creamy Crispy Paneer Kebabs

Serve: 1

Prep: 10 min Cook: 10 min

Ingredients and Quantity

- 3.5 oz Verka Paneer (chopped into thick slices)
- 0.88 oz Flaxseed powder
- 2 tbsp Coconut milk
- 3 tsp Ghee
- 1 tbsp Mint chutney
- Salt and pepper to taste

Directions:

- Spread mint chutney on one side of the paneer pieces and make a sandwich.

2. Mix together the salt, pepper and flax seed powder in a bowl.

3. Dip the paneer in the coconut milk and then dredge in the flax powder.

4. Place on the grill pan of the air fryer and cook until done, flipping once in between.

Fried Aubergine

Serve: 3

Prep: 10 min Cook: 10 min

Ingredients and Quantity

- 1 Aubergine (cut into slices)
- 1 tsp Garam masala powder
- 1 tsp Red chili powder
- ½ tsp Roasted fennel powder
- ½ tsp Turmeric powder
- 2 tsp Olive oil
- Salt to taste

Directions:

- Season the eggplant pieces with turmeric-salt mixture on both sides and place aside for 10 minutes.

2. Mix together the rest of the ingredients except the oil and coat the aubergine slices with it.

3. Preheat the air fryer to 360 degrees Fahrenheit for 10 minutes.

4. Brush oil on the aubergine slices and cook in the air fryer for 10 minutes.

5. Serve and enjoy

Stuffed Mushrooms

Serve: 3

Prep: 10 min Cook: 10 min

Ingredients and Quantity

- 3 Portobello mushrooms (stems removed)
- 1 Tomato (diced)
- 1 Green bell pepper (diced)
- 2 Ham slices (chopped fine)
- 1 tsp Garlic (minced)
- 1 Red onion (diced)
- ½ tsp Truffle salt
- Black pepper Just a dash
- 1 tbsp Olive oil
- Grated Cheddar cheese as desired

Directions:

- Preheat the air fryer to 320 degrees Fahrenheit for 10 minutes. Coat the mushrooms with oil.

2. Mix together the rest of the ingredients in a bowl and stuff it into the mushroom caps.

3. Air fry for around 8 minutes and serve once done.

Cauliflower Steak

Serve: 3

Prep: 10 min Cook: 30 min

Ingredients and Quantity

- 1 Purple cauliflower head (sliced carefully)
- Olive oil Just for drizzling
- Salt to taste
- ½ Bell pepper (thinly sliced)
- ½ Yellow onion (thinly sliced)
- Old Bay seasoning to taste
- 1 tbsp Olive oil

Directions:

- Drizzle oil on the cauliflower and then season it with salt and Old Bay seasoning.

2. Place in the baking dish and sprinkle the bell pepper and onion over.

3. Bake for 25 minutes in an oven preheated to 375 degrees Fahrenheit.

4. Transfer into an air fryer at 360 degrees Fahrenheit for 3 minutes until lightly charred.

5. Serve and enjoy

Stuffed Crab

Serve: 3

Prep: 10 min Cook: 20 min

Ingredients and Quantity

- 3 Small crabs (steamed, meat removed)
- 1 Garlic clove (chopped)
- 1 Red onion (chopped)
- Zero Cuisine
- 4 tbsp Cauliflower Mash powder
- 1 Egg
- 1 cup Cauliflower (chopped)
- 1 tbsp White onion (chopped)
- 1 tbsp Olive oil

Directions:

- Heat oil in a pan and sauté the red onion and garlic in it.

2. Add the crab meat and half the cauliflower mash and mix well. Remove from the flame.

3. Mix the rest of the cauliflower mash in a little water to make a paste. Add the egg to the paste and mix well.

4. Stuff the crab meat mixture back into the crab and coat the crabs with the egg mix. Air fry until golden brown.

5. Microwave the cauliflower for 1 minute and the sauté the cauliflower and white onion in a pan, seasoning it with salt and pepper.

6. Serve the cauliflower couscous with the stuffed crabs.

Cheesy Scrambled Eggs

Serve: 2

Prep: 2 min Cook: 10 min

Ingredients and Quantity

- 2 Large eggs
- 4/5 cup Almond Milk
- 1 ¾ oz Grated cheese
- 8 Cherry tomatoes (halved)
- Salt and pepper to taste

Directions:

- Lightly coat the air fryer paddle with some oil spray. Place the paddle in the machine.

2. Whisk together the milk and eggs with salt and pepper in a bowl and cook it in the air fryer, ensuring the lid is closed firmly. Cook for 6 minutes.

3. Open the lid; scrape the egg mix from the bowl sides and the mix in the tomatoes. Cook for 3 more minutes.

4. Sprinkle the grated cheese over the egg and leave to melt for around 30 seconds.

5. Serve and enjoy

Chicken in Screw Pine Leaves

Serve: 4

Prep: 10 min Cook: 15 min

Ingredients and Quantity

- 17 ½ oz Chicken breast (chopped into medium pieces)
- 1 Shallot
- 2 tsp Turmeric
- Salt and pepper to taste

Directions:

- Mix all the ingredients together and leave the chicken to marinate overnight refrigerated.

2. Roll a screw pine leave around each piece of chicken and seal with a toothpick.

3. Spray some olive oil over the air fryer basket. Cook for 15 minutes at 360 degrees Fahrenheit.

4. Serve and enjoy

Tilapia Salad

Serve: 2

Prep: 5 min Cook: 15-18 min

Ingredients and Quantity

- 6 cups Mixed greens
- 1 cup Cherry tomatoes
- 1/3 cup Red onion (diced)
- 1 Avocado (sliced
- Tortilla crusted tilapia fillets (frozen)
- ½ cup Chipotle-lime dressing

Directions:

- Drizzle oil on both sides of the fish filets. Cook for 15-18 minutes at 390 degrees Fahrenheit.

2. Distribute the rest of the ingredients between two bowls and toss.

3. Add the cooked fish filets and serve.

Spicy Chicken Wings

Serve: 4

Prep: 5 min Cook: 30 min

Ingredients and Quantity

- 2 lbs Chicken wings
- Salt and pepper to taste
- 1 tbsp Vegetable oil
- 1 ½ tbsp Buffalo sauce

Directions:

- Toss the chicken wings in salt, pepper and oil. Cook for 25 minutes in an air fryer.

2. Add the buffalo sauce over the chicken and cook for another 3 minutes.

3. Serve and enjoy

Prawns in Creamy Garlic Sauce

Serve: 5

Prep: 10 min Cook: 4 min

Ingredients and Quantity

- 10 Shrimps

Sauce:

- 3 Garlic cloves (minced)
- ¾ oz Butter
- 2/3 cup Thick cream
- Salt and pepper to taste
- 1 tsp Lemon juice
- ½ tsp Lemon zest
- 1 tbsp Vegetable oil

- 1 ½ tbsp Buffalo sauce

Directions:

- Combine all the sauce ingredients in a saucepan and simmer on low flame. Leave aside.

2. Discard the antennae, telson, walking legs, intestine and rostrum of the shrimps and slit the meat lengthwise.

3. Season the shrimps with salt and pepper, drizzling some oil over them. Pass a skewer through lengthwise.

4. Cook for 4 minutes in an air fryer at 360 degrees Fahrenheit.

5. Serve with the garlic sauce.

Roasted Pork belly

Serve: 6

Prep: 10 min Cook: 5 hours

Ingredients and Quantity

- 24 ½ oz Pork belly
- 2 tsp Garlic salt
- 1 tsp Five spice powder
- 1 tsp Ground white pepper
- Salt to taste
- 2 tbsp Lime juice

Directions:

- Cook the pork belly in water for 3-4 hours.

2. Discard the water and leave to dry for 3 hours.

3. Score the pork skin using a knife and massage the rest of the ingredients into it.

4. Preheat the air fryer to 320 degrees Fahrenheit for 10 minutes.

5. Cook the pork belly for 30 minutes skin side up in the air fryer.

6. Cook for another 30 minutes at 360 degrees Fahrenheit.

7. Serve and enjoy

Crispy Kale

Serve: 3

Prep: 5 min Cook: 3 minutes

Ingredients and Quantity

- 1 bunch Fresh kale torn into pieces)
- Salt to taste
- Olive oil for spraying

Directions:

- Preheat the air fryer for 5 minutes at 360 degrees Fahrenheit. Spread the kale in the air fryer basket and spray oil over.

2. Air fry for 2-3 minutes until crispy, ensuring to check in between.

3. Season with salt and serve.

Cheesy Broccoli

Serve: 2-4

Prep: 10 min Cook: 15 min

Ingredients and Quantity

- 2 pounds Broccoli florets
- 2 tbsp Olive oil
- 1 tsp Kosher salt
- ½ tsp Ground black pepper
- 1/3 cup Kalamata olives (halved, pitted)
- 2 tsp Lemon zest (grated)
- ¼ cup Parmesan cheese (shaved)

Directions:

- Boil water in a saucepan and cook the broccoli in it for 3-4 minutes. Drain.

2. Toss the broccoli with salt, pepper and oil. Place in the air fryer basket and cook for 15 minutes at 400 degrees Fahrenheit, tossing twice in between.

3. Transfer to a serving bowl and toss in the lemon zest, olives and cheese.

4. Serve and enjoy

Salmon with Almond Crust

Serve: 3

Prep: 5 min Cook: 20 min

Ingredients and Quantity

- 3 Wild caught salmon
- Pesto as required
- Salt and pepper to taste
- Almonds (ground) as required

Directions:

- Marinate the fish with the pesto, salt and pepper for an hour.

2. Air fry for 20 minutes, flipping midway.

3. Serve sprinkled with the ground almonds.

Balsamic Broccoli

Serve: 3

Prep: 5 min Cook: 8 min

Ingredients and Quantity

- 2 Broccoli bunch (chopped into pieces)
- 1 tbsp Olive oil
- 1 tbsp Honey
- 2 tbsp Balsamic vinegar

Directions:

- Preheat the air fryer to 372 degrees Fahrenheit. Toss together the broccoli and olive oil.

2. Air fry for 8 minutes, tossing midway.

3. Mix together the vinegar and honey and toss the broccoli in it.

4. Serve and enjoy

Beef Steak

Serve: 4

Prep: 10 min Cook: 14 min

Ingredients and Quantity:

- 1 tbsp Olive oil
- 2 pounds Rib eye steak
- 1 tbsp Steak rub

Directions:

- Preheat the air fryer to 400 degrees Fahrenheit for 4 minutes. Season the steak with the steak rub and brush with some olive oil.

2. Cook for 14 minutes, flipping the steak half way through.

3. Serve and enjoy

Mini Lamb Rump Roast

Serve: 3

Prep: 5 min Cook: 20 min

Ingredients and Quantity:

- 21 oz Lamb rump
- 6 Garlic cloves (crushed)
- 2 sprigs Rosemary
- 2 tsp Olive oil

Directions:

- Rub the lamb with the garlic, oil and rosemary.

2. Place in an air fryer at 360 degrees Fahrenheit and cook for 20 minutes.

3. Serve and enjoy

Lamb Chops

Serve: 4

Prep: 15 min Cook: 22 min

Ingredients and Quantity

- 3 tbsp Olive oil
- 1 Garlic bulb
- 1 tbsp Fresh oregano (chopped finely)
- Salt and pepper to taste
- 8 Lamb chops

Directions:

- Preheat the air fryer to 392 degrees Fahrenheit. Toss the garlic with oil and cook in the air fryer basket for 12 minutes.

2. Mix together the herbs, pepper, salt and olive oil and marinate the lamb chops with half tablespoon of it for 5 minutes. Remove the garlic and place aside.

3. Add the lamb chops to the basket and cook for 5 minutes.

4. Squeeze the garlic into the remaining herb oil, season with some salt and pepper and mix well.

5. Serve the chops and the herb-garlic sauce.

Balsamic Brussels Sprouts

Serve: 3

Prep: 5 min Cook: 10 min

Ingredients and Quantity

- 2 cups Fresh Brussels sprouts (tough leaves discarded, halved)
- ¼ tsp Sea salt
- 1 tbsp Balsamic vinegar
- 1 tbsp Maple Syrup

Directions:

- Toss the Brussels sprouts with the salt, maple syrup and vinegar.

2. Place the sprouts in an air fryer basket at 400 degrees Fahrenheit for 8-10 minutes.

3. Serve and enjoy

Cajun Seasoned Salmon

Serve: 1

Prep: 5 min Cook: 7 min

Ingredients and Quantity

- 1 Fresh salmon filet
- Cajun seasoning sufficient to coat
- Lemon juice of ¼ lemon

Directions:

- Preheat the air fryer to 360 degrees Fahrenheit. Coat the salmon with the Cajun seasoning.

2. Place on the air fryer grill pan, skin side up and cook for 7 minutes.

3. Squeeze lemon juice over it and serve.

Garlic Flavored Mushroom

Serve: 4

Prep: 10 min Cook: 30 min

Ingredients and Quantity

- 1 tbsp Duck fat
- 2 pound Mushrooms (washed, dried, quartered)
- ½ tsp Garlic powder
- 2 tsp Herbes de Provence
- 2 tbsp White vermouth

Directions:

- Put the Herbes de Provence, duck fat and garlic powder in an air fryer pan and heat for 2 minutes.

2. Add in the mushrooms. Cook for around 25 minutes.

3. Mix in the vermouth and cook for an additional 5 minutes.

Cauliflower Bites

Serve: 1

Prep: 10 min Cook: 5 min

Ingredients and Quantity

- 1 ½ cups Cauliflower florets (sliced)
- 1 tbsp Olive oil
- Salt and pepper to taste

Directions:

- Preheat the air fryer to 390 degrees Fahrenheit. Toss together all the ingredients in a bowl.

2. Transfer into the air fryer basket and cook for 5-6 minutes.

3. Serve and enjoy

Shrimps Wrapped in Bacon

Serve: 3

Prep: 10 min Cook: 5-7 min

Ingredients and Quantity

- 9 Bacon slice
- 9 Shrimps

Directions:

- Preheat the air fryer to 390 degrees Fahrenheit.

2. Wrap each prawn in a bacon slice and seal with a toothpick. Refrigerate for 20 minutes.

3. Transfer into the air fryer basket and cook for 5-7 minutes.

4. Serve and enjoy

Veggie Mix

Serve: 2-4

Prep: 10 min Cook: 35 min

Ingredients and Quantity:

- 1 lb Zucchini (chopped into half-moons)

- 1 ib Yellow squash (chopped into half-moons)
- ½ ib Carrots (peeled, cubed)
- 6 tsp Olive oil
- 1 tsp Kosher salt
- ½ tsp Ground white pepper
- 1 tbsp Tarragon leaves (roughly chopped)

Directions:

- Toss the carrots with 2 teaspoons oil and place in an air fryer basket.

2. Cook for 5 minutes at 400 degrees Fahrenheit. Toss the zucchini and squash in the rest of the oil, salt and pepper and place in an air fryer.

3. Cook for 30 minutes, tossing thrice in between. Toss with the tarragon.

4. Serve and enjoy

Conclusion

This book Clean Keto Air Fryer Cookbook will guide on how to live and maintain a clean keto lifestyle. Over 500 recipes were feature in this book to help you pass through ketosis and lose weight drastically.

Part 2

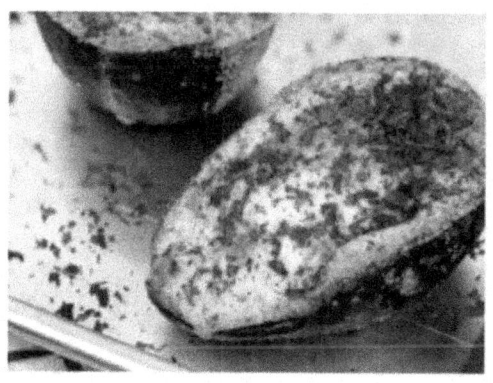

Baked Avocado Egg

Did you know that avocado is a fruit, not a vegetable? Avocado is considered the "fruit" of the tree! Avocados are bursting with nutrients that are great to incorporate into your daily diet. From a good guacamole to avocado toast, and now these tasty baked avocado eggs. You can find tons of recipes to use avocado, so you don't get bored of them.

Ingredients

1 Avocados Large

2 Eggs Small

Salt And Pepper To Taste

1/4 Cup Shredded Cheddar Optional

1 T Fresh Parsley

Instructions

Preheat air fryer to 400.

Cut avocados in half and remove the seed

Place avocados face up on cutting board.

Crack 1 egg into the avocado; make sure to keep the yolk intact.

Air-Fry for 12-15 minutes or until eggs are desired temperature.

Sprinkle with optional cheese.

Scotch Eggs with Spicy Pepper Sauce

Prep Time 20 mins| Cook Time 25 mins |Total Time 45 mins

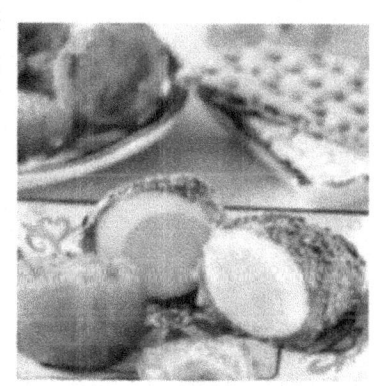

Love scotch eggs but hate all the extra fat that comes with frying them? This Air Fried Scotch Eggs give you all the great flavor of traditional scotch eggs without all of extra grease and fat since they're made in your Air Fryer.

Ingredients

1 Pound Bulk Pork Sausage

1 Tablespoon Finely Chopped Fresh Chives

2 Tablespoons Finely Chopped Fresh Parsley

1/8 Teaspoon Freshly Grated Nutmeg

1/8 Teaspoon Salt

1/8 Teaspoon Ground Black Pepper

4 Hard-Cooked Eggs Peeled

1 Cup Shredded Parmesan Cheese

2 Teaspoons Coarse-Ground Mustard

Instructions

For the eggs: In a large bowl combine sausage, mustard, chives, parsley, nutmeg, salt, and black pepper. Gently mix until everything is well combined. Shape mixture into four equal-size patties.

Please each egg on a sausage patty and shape sausage around egg. Dip each in shredded Parmesan cheese to cover completely, pressing lightly to adhere. Make sure the cheese shreds are well-pressed into the meat, so that they do not fly around in the air fryer.

Arrange eggs in air fryer basket. Spray lightly with nonstick vegetable oil. Set fryer to 400°F for 15 minutes. Halfway through cook time, turn eggs and spray with vegetable oil.

Serve with coarse-ground mustard.

Easy Frittata Breakfast

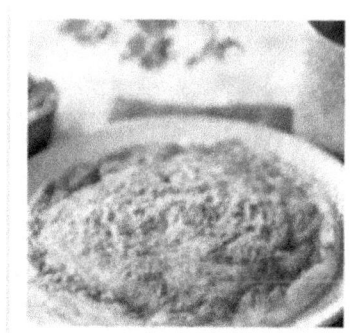

Ingredients:

3 eggs

½ Italian sausage

4 cherry tomatoes (in half)

1 tablespoon olive oil

Chopped parsley

Grano Padano cheese (or parmesan)

Salt/Pepper

INSTRUCTIONS:

Preheat the Air Fryer to 360 degrees

Place the cherry tomatoes and sausage in the baking accessory and bake at 360 degrees for 5 minutes.

In a small bowl, whisk the remaining ingredients together.

Remove the baking accessory from the Air Fryer and add the egg mixture, making sure it is even. Bake for another 5 minutes.

White Bean Toasts with Burst Grape Tomatoes and Pancetta

Serves: 4

-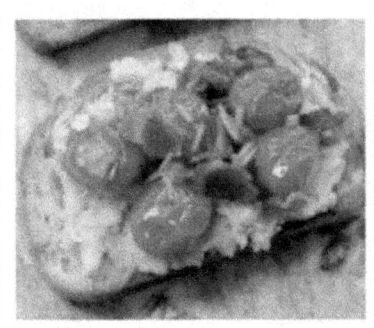

Ingredients

8 Ounces Pancetta

1 Cup Grape Tomatoes

1 (15-Ounce) Can Cannellini Beans, Drained And Rinsed

1 To 2 Tablespoons Olive Oil

1 Tablespoon Chopped Fresh Rosemary

Salt And Freshly Ground Black Pepper

4 Slices Thick-Sliced Ciabatta Bread

Chopped Fresh Chives

Instructions

Pre-heat the air fryer to 400°F.

Cut the pancetta into ½-inch cubes and toss them into the air fryer basket. Air-fry at 400ºF for 8 minutes. Give the air fryer basket a shake and toss in the grape tomatoes. Air-fry for another 5 to 7 minutes, until the skin on the tomatoes just starts to burst open and the pancetta is crispy. (Alternatively you can cook the pancetta in a sauté pan on the stovetop. Add the grape tomatoes when the pancetta just starts to brown and cook the two together for a few more minutes until the skin on the tomatoes just starts to burst open.) Set the pancetta and tomatoes aside.

Place the cannellini beans and olive oil in a large bowl. Smash the beans with the back of a fork until they are coarsely mashed, stir in the rosemary and season to taste with salt and freshly ground black pepper.

Brush the bread slices generously with olive oil and place them in the air fryer. Air-fry at 400ºF for 5 minutes, turning them over for even browning. (If you are making this on the stovetop, heat a large sauté pan over medium-high heat. Drizzle with olive oil to coat the bottom of the pan. Fry the bread slices on both sides until toasted and light brown, adding more oil as needed.)

Assemble the toasts by first spreading some of the mashed cannellini bean mixture on each toasted slice. Top with some pancetta and burst tomatoes, season with a couple twists of freshly ground black pepper and garnish with fresh chopped chives. Serve warm or at room temperature a slice as an appetizer or cut into triangles to serve as hors d'ouevres.

Loaded Cauliflower Hashbrowns

Serves: 8

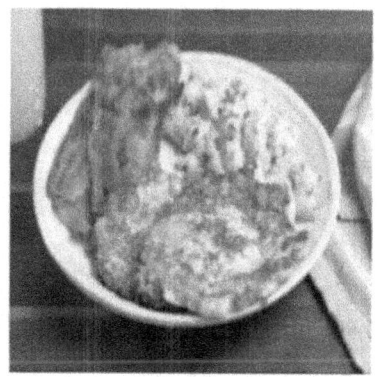

Everyone loves a hashbrown for breakfast, but wait until you taste a cauliflower hashbrown – a little lighter but full of flavor!

Ingredients

4 Slices Thick-Cut Bacon, Diced

1 Head Of Cauliflower

½ Cup Finely Diced Onion

½ Cup Finely Diced Red And Green Bell Pepper

1 Egg

½ Cup Chickpea, Almond, Or All-Purpose Flour

1 Cup Grated Cheddar Cheese

½ Teaspoon Paprika

1 Teaspoon Salt

Freshly Ground Black Pepper

Instructions

Pre-heat the air fryer to 400°F.

Air-fry the bacon and onion for 8 to 10 minutes, until the bacon is crispy, shaking the basket a few times during the cooking process. (Add a little water to the air fryer drawer if the bacon grease starts to smoke.)

Grate the head of cauliflower with a box grater or finely chop it in a food processor. You should have about 3½ cups. Place the cauliflower in the center of a clean kitchen towel and twist it to squeeze all the water out. (This can be done in two batches to make it easier to drain all the water from the cauliflower.)

Place the cauliflower in a large bowl and add the bacon, onions, peppers, egg, flour, Cheddar cheese, paprika, salt and pepper. Mix until well combined. Shape the mixture into 8 oval shaped patties and freeze for at least 1 hour.

Pre-heat air fryer to 400°F.

Spray or brush the air fryer basket with a little oil. Air-fry the hash browns in batches for 10 minutes, turning them over halfway through the cooking process. Season with salt and freshly ground black pepper.

Deep Dish Prosciutto, Spinach & Mushroom Pizza - Air Fryer Version

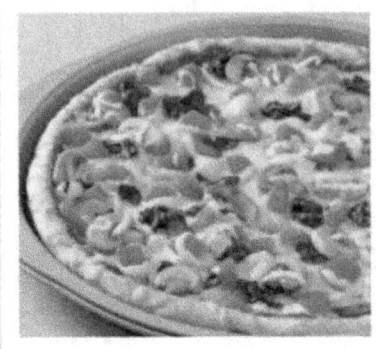

Prep time: 20 mins | Cook time: 35 mins | Total time: 55 mins

Serves: 2

It is critical when using your air fryer for this recipe to find the right sized pan. Make sure your pan fits into your air fryer basket before you start or you'll be very disappointed.

Ingredients

3 Ounces Button Mushrooms, Sliced

½ Cup Frozen Spinach, Thawed

1 Tablespoon Olive Oil

¼ Teaspoon Italian Seasoning

12 Ounces Pizza Dough

⅓ Cup Pizza Sauce

1½ Cups Grated Mozzarella Cheese

3 Ounces Thinly Sliced Prosciutto

Instructions

Toss the mushrooms with the olive oil and Italian seasoning, and set aside to marinate for at least 15 minutes. Squeeze as much liquid as possible from the spinach and set the spinach aside as well.

Pre-heat air fryer to 370"F.

Grease the inside of a 7-inch baking pan with olive oil, or use a pan with a non-stick surface. Roll or stretch the pizza dough out into a circle that is 8 to 9 inches in diameter and transfer it to the pan, pressing the crust up the sides of the pan. Dock the dough by piercing holes in the bottom crust with a fork. Transfer the pan to the air fryer basket.

Air-fry at 370ºF for 5 minutes. Remove the pan from the air fryer. Flip the crust over in the pan by inverting it onto a plate and sliding it back into the pan. (Yes, this seems counterintuitive and you will worry about the walls of the pizza collapsing, but they won't.) Return the pan to the air fryer and air-fry for 5 minutes to brown the bottom of the crust. Flip the crust back over in the pan.

Fill the inside of the pizza crust with the sauce and top with half of the mozzarella cheese. Layer half of the spinach and mushrooms over the cheese. Repeat with another layer of cheese and another layer of spinach and mushrooms. Tear the prosciutto up into pieces and scatter the pieces on top of the pizza. Return the pan to the air fryer.

Air-fry at 350°F for 10 to 12 minutes until crust is brown and the cheese has melted.

Serve with a nice salad and a glass of red wine!

A Monte Cristo sandwich is a "French toasted ham and cheese sandwich". It has the sweet taste of French toast with the salty flavor of the ham and Swiss cheese to make a pretty divine combination.

Monte Cristo Sandwich

Serves: 1

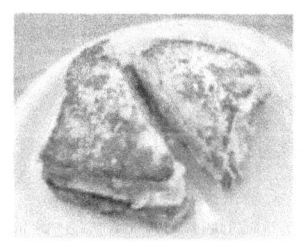

Ingredients

1 Egg

3 Tablespoons Half And Half

¼ Teaspoon Vanilla Extract

2 Slices Sourdough, White Or Multigrain Bread

2½ Ounces Sliced Swiss Cheese

2 Ounces Slices Deli Ham

2 Ounces Sliced Deli Turkey

1 Teaspoon Butter, Melted

Powdered Sugar

Instructions

Combine the egg, half and half and vanilla extract in a shallow bowl.

Place the bread on the counter. Build a sandwich with one slice of Swiss cheese, the ham, the turkey and then a second slice of Swiss cheese on one slice of the bread. Top with the other slice of bread and press down slightly to flatten.

Pre-heat the air fryer to 350ºF.

Cut out a piece of aluminum foil about the same size as the bread and brush the foil with melted butter. Dip both sides of the sandwich in the egg batter. Let the batter soak into bread for about 30 seconds on each side. Then place the sandwich on the greased aluminum foil and transfer it to the air fryer basket. For extra browning, brush the top of the sandwich with melted butter. Air-fry at 350ºF for 10 minutes. Flip the sandwich over, brush with butter and air-fry for an additional 8 minutes.

Transfer the sandwich to a serving plate and sprinkle with powdered sugar. Serve with raspberry or blackberry preserves on the side.

Keto Creamed Spinach

Prep Time 10 mins | Cook Time 15 mins | Total Time 25 mins

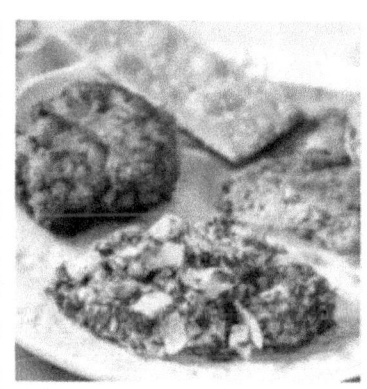

This Keto Creamed Spinach recipe is the perfect quick and easy side dish for most any entree! It's creamy, low carb and made in no time in your air fryer.

Ingredients

1 10 Ounce Package Frozen Spinach Thawed

1/2 Cup Chopped Onion

2 Teaspoons Minced Garlic

4 Ounces Cream Cheese Diced

1 Teaspoon Pepper

1 Teaspoon Salt

1/2 Teaspoon Ground Nutmeg

1/4 Cup Shredded Parmesan Cheese

Instructions

Grease a 6 inch pan and set aside.

In the medium bowl, combine spinach, onion, garlic, cream cheese dices, salt, pepper, and nutmeg. Pour into greased pan.

Set air fryer to 350°F for 10 minutes. Open and stir the spinach to mix the cream cheese through the spinach.

Sprinkle the Parmesan cheese on top. Set air fryer to 400°F for 5 minutes or until the cheese has melted and browned.

www.ingramcontent.com/pod-product-compliance
Lightning Source LLC
Chambersburg PA
CBHW071437070526
44578CB00001B/112